MW01634011

Praise for this Book

Paddy Kamen distils several years of personal exploration and direct experience in the world of neuroscience to bring us a book as illuminating as it is practical. Using refreshingly lucid prose, Kamen filters a complex network of knowledge in brief, to-the-point chapters that can be picked up and meaningfully savored in our all-too-brief leisure time. But don't be fooled — within these invitational snippets Kamen opens windows to a wealth of knowledge and practical possibility to the earnest seeker of life-altering, brain-enhancing technologies.

Dr. Susan Cheshire Brown
Co-Founder of NeurOptimal® Dynamical
Neurofeedback Systems

This exciting book about improving one's brain is understandable, practical, motivating. If you weren't reading the scientific literature, this is what you missed. If you were, you were taking notes. Don't bother looking for them. The information is captured here on pages that will grab you at the beginning and hold your attention right to the end.

Claudia L. Osborn, DO, FACOI
Author of *Over My Head: A Doctor's Story of Head Injury
From The Inside Looking Out*

The best of the West (science) and the best of the East (meditation) have begun a mating dance in our time. It's impossible to predict what wondrous offspring this union may produce but, whether they realize it or not, every human has a stake in this courtship. Kamen's book is an effective antidote to pessimism. Better Brain Better Life implies the realistic possibility of a dramatically better world for everyone, and relatively soon.

Shinzen Young
Vipassana/Mindfulness Meditation Teacher
Author of *Natural Pain Relief: How to Soothe & Dissolve Physical Pain with Mindfulness*
and *The Science Of Enlightenment* (audio)

Paddy Kamen understands that the brain is the most plastic organ in the body. In her book, she meticulously explores the world of innovative and alternative brain interventions that are designed to heal, maximize intelligence and enhance the capacity to learn. This book delivers a message of hope and happiness to everyone.

Donalee Markus, Ph.D.
Founder of Designs for Strong Minds
Author of *Retrain Your Business Brain*

This is a special book for all of us on a brain journey – and we all are on our own personal brain journey. Paddy Kamen hits the highlights of the most meaningful of all the sciences – brain science – with an accent on brain regeneration and growth through lifestyle strategies, and the avoidance of brain tissue loss through exposure to toxins, which are all too common. It is well-researched, touches on the latest techniques and interesting studies and researchers. Reading this book will expand your cortex, guaranteed!

Peter H. Dohan, M.D.
Diplomate American Board of Pathology (retired)
Dr. Dohan practiced surgical and clinical pathology with a great interest, both personal and familial, in brain science.

Paddy Kamen has done a wonderful job of integrating and highlighting a great deal of information about brainwave training and she presents it in an easy-to-assimilate manner. It is evident that she has personally experienced the extensive use of many of the neurofeedback systems in this exciting field. This alone eminently qualifies her to author this interesting survey of this promising field.

Les Fehmi, Ph.D.
Co-author with Jim Robbins of
The Open-Focus Brain and *Dissolving Pain*

iv

Better Brain Better Life captured me with its engaging explanations of the most interesting features and interpretations of the many facets of brain-mind-spirit interaction. Paddy Kamen skillfully describes the essential messages embedded in various scenarios lived by real people who either experienced brain injury, developed instrumentation for measuring or modifying brain activity, or in some way contributed ideas to reveal how the brain works in ways that relate to how we live. You will be glad you found such an entertaining and educational gem.

Gerald P. Kozlowski, Ph.D.
BCN-Certified Fellow in EEG biofeedback (BCIA)
Psychophysiology Faculty, University of Natural Medicine

Check Out These Tips for Brain Enhancement

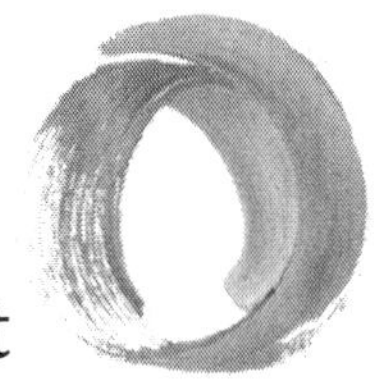

Better Brain Better Life

Tips and Tales
From the Tantalizing World
of Brain Science

Paddy Kamen

Copyright © 2013, Paddy Kamen

All Rights Reserved

Published by Better Brain Publishing

Kelowna, British Columbia, Canada

All rights reserved. No part of this book may be transmitted or reproduced in any form, or by any electronic or mechanical means, including information storage and retrieval systems, without written permission of the above publisher of the book, except in the case of a reviewer who may quote brief passages in a review or certain other non-commercial uses permitted by copyright law. For permissions email: info@betterbrainbetterlife.com.

For additional information, please visit: www.betterbrainbetterlife.com

Library and Archives Canada Cataloguing in Publication
    Kamen, Paddy
    Better Brain Better Life: Tips and Tales from the Tantalizing World of Brain Science
    Paddy Kamen.
Includes bibliographical references.
ISBN 978-0-9880178-0-1
Issued also in electronic format: ISBN 978-0-9880178-1-8

1. Self-actualization (psychology)
2. Brain Health (self-help)
3. Brain Research (psychology)
4. Meditation (self-help/psychology)

DISCLAIMER: This book and the information contained in it, is sold with the understanding that the author and publisher are not engaged in giving professional advice. The author and publisher specifically disclaim any liability that is incurred from the use or application of the contents of this book. All content herein is provided for informational purposes only and should not be misconstrued as medical advice. Readers should visit a qualified health care professional for all their health care needs.

Editing: JoAnne Sommers, Cherie F. Hanson, Raffaela Civello,
and with thanks to Gerald P. Kozlowski

Cover Design (front): Stephanie Symons
Cover Design (back): Leighan Sindrey, LS Creative Co.
Zen Circle on Cover: courtesy Debbi Lynn, www.kodachrom.com

Dedication

To my meditation teacher Shinzen Young, who is probably not waiting for me to finish the book I'm writing on him…probably never was waiting, being who he is…and who has helped me immeasurably. Shinzen is a hero of consciousness.

And to Les Fehmi, another pioneer who also helps me and my loved ones – spouse, children and grandchildren – with the practices and technologies he has created. Another hero!

Shinzen continues to be active in research on the brain and meditation, in addition to offering both online and residential retreats. Les serves local and international clients from his office in Princeton, N.J. Both have written excellent books on working with pain, among other subjects, and offer superb guidance into non-dual states of consciousness through audio recordings.

The longer I live this life the more I realize that love in action is, indeed, love itself. The actions of these men are, in their essence, a reflection of love. Their work with others allows for the arising of love and joy, deep peace and an attitude of service that spreads a fragrant essence, reaching more lives and hearts and minds than they can ever know.

They too, stand on the shoulders of giants, as do all of us who choose the path of insight, learning and love. I like the view from their shoulders and I thank them for lifting me up!

Table of Contents

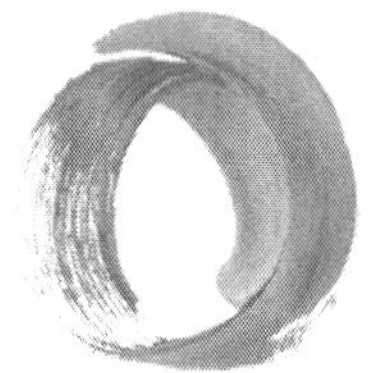

Introduction

*Buddhist practitioners familiar
with the workings of the mind
have long been aware that it
can be transformed through
training…. In a real sense the
brain we develop reflects the life
we lead.*

14th Dalai Lama

Introduction

When I was a kid, we often would quip, "you don't have to be a brain surgeon," or "it's not rocket science," indicating, with some degree of disdain, that the task at hand was not particularly difficult. Other than those off-the-cuff remarks, I never thought much about my brain or my mind until, as an adolescent, I began reading psychology and spirituality. Don't get me wrong, I didn't have a long, impressive reading list, but I did dabble in Jung and Ram Dass and the Christian mystics.

Fast forward to 2005. I was on the cusp of my 50s and frustrated because I couldn't seem to achieve my goals. Over a period of about ten years, I'd repeatedly become excited about a project, start working on it with great enthusiasm, achieve a few milestones and then, well, I'd stop. I would become alienated from the parts of me that had recently been so excited, creative and confident. I avoided taking action and sensed a huge chasm in my gut, seething with murky dread. I would simply stop doing the work that would move me toward my goals. I felt simply awful about the situation, and would distract myself to avoid the uncomfortable emotions. I couldn't get past it.

One of the blessings of my life during this time was that I had become a consistent practitioner of mindfulness meditation, which gave me access to the inner workings of my (seemingly dysfunctional) mind and emotions.

Meditation practice is akin to good talk-therapy or regular journaling in that it helps me see my self-defeating patterns of thought and action; but it is more profound than talk-therapy or journaling because it actually changes my brain (see Chapters 2, 13 & 22). I'm no longer just "cogitating" about my world and experiences, but instead I practice noticing the spaces between thoughts, really feeling the emotions in the body rather than suppressing them, and repeatedly severing the link between thought and emotion, thereby starving both of the energy that keeps me trapped. I'm learning, through fits and starts, that this leads to a new kind of freedom.

It was also around this time that I learned about brain enhancement through neurofeedback: biofeedback for the brain. Twenty sessions with this technology, administered by a neuropsychologist, improved my cognitive and behavioral functioning to an amazing degree: I was happier, spontaneously thankful, able to multi-task with ease, and mentally sharper. I was so excited about this transformation that I felt called to find a way to keep learning about brain enhancement and to make a contribution to the field.

Brain science today is, in my view, a contender for the field of study that holds the greatest hope for humanity. In fact, the "looking in" of brain research, in a strange way mirrors the "looking out" of astronomy, for, as Gerald M. Edelman points out in *Bright Air, Brilliant Fire: On The Matter of the Mind,* there are more synapses in the average brain than there are positively charged particles in the known universe.

My meditation teacher, Shinzen Young, is involved in research at Harvard Medical School that aims to map the meditative mind. The research being conducted in collaboration with David Vago and the Functional Neuroimaging Laboratory aims to uncover the neural correlates of distinct modalities of awareness that are described in Shinzen's Basic Mindfulness System. Through their continued work together, Shinzen and David are also aiming to capture the experience of cessation, a deep subjective state of mental quiescence in which there is a complete absence of all craving and ignorance. Also described as enlightenment, these deep and subtle meditative states have yet to be paired at both a phenomenological and neurobiological level. Imagine the possibilities for personal, political and social change as science finds ways for more of us to easily experience the oneness of all life and the stillness that underlies thought.

And so I find "tantalizing" to be just the right word to describe the latest discoveries of brain science research, and, while some of this research might be beyond the average reader, much of it can impact individual lives here and now in ways that are highly significant. For example, in this book you can read about dietary supplements that improve cognition and memory; herbs that aid in stroke recovery; how a rocking motion improves sleep; how mindfulness meditation grows grey matter in the brain; how weight training improves cognition; and why avoiding dietary gluten can improve outcomes for schizophrenics. This is practical research indeed.

This book represents a significantly happy moment for me as I fulfill my desire to share my research with other non-scientists, and I hope it will open new vistas of interest and perhaps even personal change for you. One thing is certain: we don't need to be rocket scientists or brain surgeons to understand most of what science is revealing about our amazing brains and our incredible capacity for learning and growth. I'm applying much of what I have learned about the brain in my own life and it has made a tremendous difference, including helping me to break through those old fears and manifest my dreams.

It is an exciting time to be alive. There are many pioneers in brain research around the world who are discovering new ways for us to embrace the potential inherent in being alive. Some of them are covered in this book. I celebrate their work, for they are true heroes, venturing into the unknown to bring back precious knowledge that leads us toward a new understanding of what it means to be human.

Paddy Kamen

British Columbia
Canada

Chapter 1

Turmeric Seasons Brain Science

Brain science is becoming deliciously spicy. Turmeric long cherished as a culinary seasoning in India, Persia, Malaysia and Thailand, has been found to contain an amazing compound that helps to protect and regenerate brain cells after the devastating effects of stroke.

The Neurology Laboratory at the Salk Institute for Biological Studies, Cedars-Sinai Medical Center in Los Angeles, was the scene of this remarkable discovery, and Paul A. Lapchak, Ph.D. was the study's lead investigator. Lapchak is a brain science researcher with 12 years' experience in the field of strokes. Prior to that he worked on Alzheimer's and Parkinson's diseases.

In an interview with BetterBrainBetterLife.com, Lapchak revealed: "We knew that curcumin, the chemical component of turmeric, has shown an effect in stroke research. Our concern is that it takes a long time to get into the brain and doesn't reach its target in high concentrations. Time is of the essence with stroke treatment and we needed to find a way to get the high-dose benefits of curcumin into the brain quickly."

Lapchak and his colleagues did just that, creating a curcumin-hybrid compound – CNB-001 – through a laborious trial-and-error process. Fortunately, the compound repairs stroke damage at the molecular level. As Lapchak explains, "CNB-001 has many of the same benefits as curcumin but appears to be a better choice of compound for acute stroke because it crosses the blood-brain barrier, is quickly distributed in the brain, and moderates several critical mechanisms involved in neuronal survival."

We needed to find a way to get the high-dose benefits of curcumin into the brain quickly.

As stated in the Cedars-Sinai news release: "When brain tissue is deprived of blood and oxygen, a cascading series of interrelated events triggers at the molecular level, breaking down the normal electrical and chemical signaling pathways responsible for nourishing and supporting neurons. The environment quickly becomes toxic, killing brain cells and destroying their support structures."

CNB-001 appears to work by interrupting this destruction. In animal models it prevented cell death and, most importantly, reduced memory problems and the physical challenges of muscle and movement control. It proved to be effective when administered up to an hour after stroke.

There are two main types of stroke: ischemic (caused by a blood clot), and hemorrhagic (caused by rupture of a blood vessel). CNB-001 was used with ischemic stroke, the most prevalent form, occurring in 87 percent of all cases.

One other drug – tissue plasminogen activator (tPA) – has been proven effective in mitigating the results of an ischemic stroke.

The drug tPA is approved for intravenous injection to dissolve clots and reinstate blood flow. If blood and oxygen are restored in time, the consequences of stroke, such as impairment to functionality in speech, memory, and movement may be reduced.

Lapchak says that his new compound is just as effective as tPA and could work well in concert with it. He is also excited about other uses for the compound. "It's still early days but my colleagues have found it to be very effective in Alzheimer's disease and traumatic brain injury in animal studies."

The research team led by Lapchak has now developed a second-generation compound and is hoping to move into clinical trials. "The next step is to make sure the drug is safe for use in human subjects," explains Lapchak. "And we're trying to obtain funding to develop the compound."

Does a traditional Indian diet, rich in turmeric, reduce incidence of stroke?

This research on curcumin begs the question of whether dietary consumption of turmeric, long a staple seasoning in South Asia, has salutary effects on brain health. Could consumption of turmeric in food reduce the incidence of stroke?

Lapchak reviewed the scientific literature on this question and finds that the incidence of ischemic stroke in India seems to be tied to dietary changes. He writes, "India is a country in transition from that of a 'developing' country to a 'developed' nation, and the typical consumed food has changed from a vegetarian diet with unrefined grains to refined products and high-saturated-fat and high-cholesterol-containing foods such as ghee, the clarified butter used in India."

He goes on to note a 2006 study that showed a 20-fold increase in ischemic stroke between 1969 and 1998. Lapchak posits that the increase in ischemic stroke in India is related to increased consumption of high-fat, high-cholesterol, insulin-resistant foods. But this doesn't prove that lower consumption of turmeric (in the move away from a traditional Indian diet) has raised the incidence of stroke.

Lapchak would like to see more research into the relationship between dietary consumption of curcumin and stroke. "We need a controlled population study to determine the relationship," he notes. "But with the increasing westernization of diet around the world it may be too late to find a population from which we could draw a control group that can be studied long-term."

Let's hope Lapchak and colleagues receive much-needed research funds. Faster stroke recovery will improve quality of life for victims of stroke. In the U.S. alone 795,000 people have new or recurring strokes each year and stroke-related medical costs in that country were a staggering $73.7 billion in 2010.

The final question: should concerned individuals add more turmeric to their diets or take curcumin supplements? The jury is still out on this, but as for me and my house, the answer is "yes" on both counts. And it surely doesn't hurt that curries taste delicious. But remember – when making a curry, use the individual spices to create the combination seasoning known as curry, rather than a prepared package. It will taste better and you can be sure to put in lots of turmeric. It will give your curry that beautiful yellow glow and may help your brain at the same time!

*We should use not only the
brains we have, but all that we
can borrow.*

Woodrow T. Wilson

When we change the way we pay attention, we gain the power to profoundly change the way we relate to our world on every level — physically, emotionally, mentally and spiritually.

Les Fehmi

Chapter 2

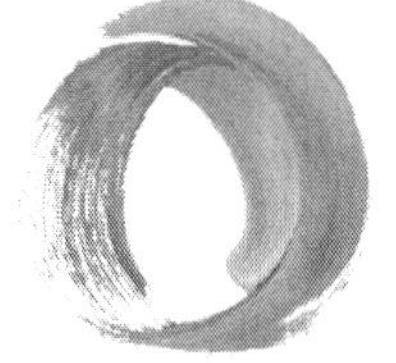

Can You Imagine? A Path to Pain Relief and Peak Performance

What if your mind was like a clear pond, and the thoughts within it darting fish that cannot disturb the surface? What if you had a sense of mental lightness even when you were really busy? What if you could dissolve any physical or emotional pain with just 30 minutes of relaxed attention?

Thanks to the pioneering work of Les Fehmi, an electrical engineer turned psychologist, thousands of people have experienced these states, and more.

Fehmi received his Ph.D. in psychology from UCLA in the late 1960s and subsequently taught at the State University of New York (SUNY) at Stony Brook. He is a pioneer in EEG technology and its application to human experience. Fehmi and Donald B. Lindsey, his mentor in graduate school, discovered how the brains of monkeys process information simultaneously at several sites – a process known as synchrony – rather than linearly, as was previously thought.

Fehmi built on his and Lindsey's synchrony discoveries and the finding of research psychologist Joe Kamiya, that profound states of mental quiet associated with alpha brainwaves could be trained with EEG-based feedback. He hooked himself up to a self-made EEG feedback device and tried to generate alpha wave activity. After 12 two-hour sessions he was getting nowhere. Then, during the 13th session, he became frustrated and gave up in abject failure. As soon as he did, the EEG showed clear and significant alpha wave activity. In fact, Fehmi experienced a profound state of consciousness that has fueled his life and work ever since.

In an interview with BetterBrainBetterLife.com Fehmi said, "That was in 1967 and I kept doing this research because I had such a powerful experience. It changed my whole being. My mind was lighter, brighter and clearer."

A key realization arising from this experience is that the way one pays attention is key to a transformed mind. Immersing and opening one's focus rather than gripping and narrowing it provides enormous benefits to the whole mind/body system. Fehmi found that severe arthritis in his hands disappeared, his personality style softened and his ability to laugh and connect with others increased. He called his system of training Open Focus™ to reflect this insight.

The next step was to find a way to help others generate alpha wave activity across the five lobes of the brain. As a professor at Stony Brook, Fehmi solicited students for research. He hooked them up to the EEG-feedback system and asked them a series of questions while he monitored their brainwaves. Asking students to imagine a dewdrop, a sunset or a beautiful flower had little effect. But when he asked them to imagine the space between their eyes their brains suddenly produced strong synchronous alpha waves. The same was true when they were asked to imagine the space between their ears. "I discovered that there is a direct relationship between imagining space and alpha," explains Fehmi.

Jim Robbins, author of *A Symphony in the Brain* (a fascinating book on the history and practice of neurofeedback explains Fehmi's discovery of the relationship between imagining space and alpha wave production thus: "When someone is looking at an object or even imagining an object, he or she is engaging many different parts of the brain to make sense of that object – via memories, senses, etc. In that state the brain is 'more desynchronized' – that is, work is occurring at different frequencies in many different parts of the brain. As soon as the eyes are closed, one is imagining space and there is a complete absence of images: the whole brain stops working hard and synchronous alpha takes over. It is a healing state, and has a powerful effect on stress."

Robbins tried many different neurofeedback systems in the course of researching his book. He recounts that after just one session with Fehmi's neurofeedback system, "I almost fell out of the chair because it was so powerful for me." Then, after using Open Focus CDs twice a day for several weeks, Robbins discovered heightened sensory awareness, greater physical relaxation and increased physical energy. He says in his book, "It was the first time in many years that I had felt so good. After a while the changes became integrated with my everyday life, so they weren't as dramatic, but there has been a marked overall improvement in the way I feel."

Given the positive changes Open Focus created in his life, Robbins became a big fan and went on to co-author Fehmi's two books: *The Open Focus Brain (2007)* and *Dissolving Pain (2010)*.

The Open Focus program has no-tech, medium-tech and high-tech solutions, suitable for everyone.

The Open Focus program consists of no-tech, medium-tech and high-tech solutions. For a no-tech experience of Open Focus one can follow instructions in Fehmi's books or work one-on-one with Fehmi, his wife and business partner Susan Shor Fehmi, MSW, or a certified Open Focus trainer. Alternately, the medium-tech solution is to use pre-recorded CDs in which Fehmi takes the listener through a variety of attention-building exercises with a focus on noticing space. The high-tech solution is Fehmi's proprietary EEG-based neurofeedback system, known as the NS-500sx. Here, five sensors are connected to a box on which a small strobe light sits. The sensors are dampened in saline solution, placed on the scalp in five places, and held there by a headband. The user puts on headphones. These convey audio feedback when one is in the brainwave state being trained for (in most cases – alpha across all lobes of the brain). The light flashes in concert with the sound, but with the eyes closed it is barely noticeable while still having an effect.

"Invitational" is a word that describes the style of guidance experienced on the Open Focus recordings, where Fehmi gently asks listeners to imagine various aspects of space within and around the body, in addition to the sense of having a body. For example: "Is it possible for you to imagine the space between your eyes?" or "Can you imagine the presence of your thumbs?" This body-centered approach places few demands on the listener by suggesting, "that no particular effort is required to listen to or follow these suggestions."

Open Focus recordings gently guide listeners to a state of focus and relaxation.

Fehmi's experiments demonstrate that alpha states have the most profound effect when they occur simultaneously over the five lobes of the brain. His system, therefore, measures activity in each lobe at the same time and gives the client positive feedback when alpha synchrony is achieved. (In contrast, many neurofeedback systems only measure brainwaves at one or two sites.) The brain teaches itself to "earn" the feedback; in other words, the learning is passive, for just as Fehmi discovered when experimenting on himself, making an effort isn't always the best way to achieve a desired result. One of the benefits of using the machine is that real time feedback on one's brainwaves can speed training.

The Princeton Biofeedback Center in Princeton, NJ is Fehmi's home base. Here, he and Shor Fehmi help clients with a wide range of challenges, including migraine headaches, mood disorders, digestive disturbances, chronic pain, asthma and ADD. They also serve the global community through Internet-based sales of training products that people can use at home.

Fehmi finds that some clients prefer the recordings, while others love the real-time feedback they receive with the neurofeedback system (the cost of these sessions may be covered by health insurance, depending on the diagnosis); still others benefit most from one-on-one verbal training. The recording options make this form of brain training readily available for most people. Results with neurofeedback are sometimes seen in just a few visits or they may take 20 or more sessions.

When asked what has most surprised him about his clinical practice with Open Focus, Fehmi responds, "It is available to everyone! When people don't get it with the home practice, then they get it with the equipment. And if they hate the equipment, they get it with the verbal one-on-one approach or with the CDs. Some are very clearly against trying the equipment and I don't push it. I let them call the shots."

Open Focus training is about attentional flexibility, that is, being able to shift one's attention from customary, culturally conditioned narrow focus to broader, more diffuse focus. Perhaps counter-intuitively, learning to relax one's focus actually enhances the ability to narrow focus when appropriate. An analogy is using muscles to lift. If one was always lifting and using one's muscles and never resting them, the ability to continue lifting would be compromised. By relaxing the muscles regularly, one ensures they will be able to do the job when called on. Besides, opening focus is inherently pleasurable because it is a form of relaxation.

Attentional training is as old as the practice of meditation training, which goes back thousands of years across all cultures and religions. Fehmi is certainly no stranger to traditional classical forms of attentional training; he has 40-plus years of Zen meditation practice under his belt. But with Open Focus he has created a completely secular approach that makes the training accessible and understandable to more people. "I wanted to find something that was secular and gave people a pure experience of mental clarity. This is what paying attention to attention has ultimately given us," he explains.

Over 70 percent of Fehmi's clients are able to dissolve physical and emotional pain.

Fehmi claims that 70–80 percent of his clients enjoy a high level of success in dissolving a number of symptoms. "With the remaining 20–30 percent there is a benefit that is not as great," he explains. "I recommend it even for people who are doing well, because they can always experience more mental clarity and relieve stress and muscle tension. We have athletes who do much better when they train their brains just before they compete. So there is a continuum from helping those with serious dysfunction all the way to optimizing functions."

As a child, Les Fehmi would imagine bringing something of great benefit to the world. He had no idea what that might be. Now in his 70s, having helped thousands of people experience clearer, lighter, brighter minds and the elimination or reduction of pain he can rest assured that he has made that contribution.

*This is my simple religion.
There is no need for temples:
no need for complicated
philosophy. Our own brain,
our own heart is our temple,
the philosophy is kindness.*
The 14th Dalai Lama

Chapter 3

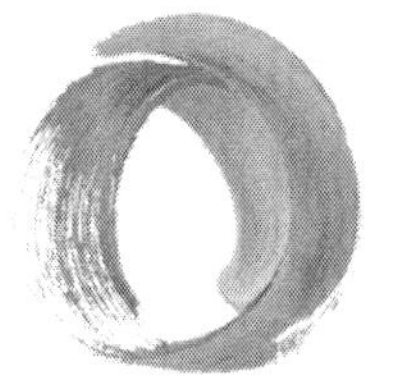

Longer DNA, Anyone?

From strengthening DNA, to improving your mental health and immune systems, science ties the ancient practice of meditation to a better life.

In a stunning research "first," the practice of meditation has been linked to cellular longevity. The discovery was made in a study that was part of the Shamatha project, which is housed within the Center for Mind and Brain at University of California, Davis (UCD).

Led by Clifford Saron, associate research scientist at the Center for Mind and Brain, the Shamatha project is one of the first long-term, detailed, matched control-group studies of the effects of intensive meditation training on mind and body.

In 2007, 30 participants took part in a three-month meditation retreat at a remote setting in Colorado, where they were instructed in mindfulness (intentionally noting thoughts and sensations in a non-judgmental way) and compassion practices by Dr. B. Alan Wallace an esteemed meditation teacher and lecturer.

Another matched group of 30 was used as a control, and then attended the retreat at a later date. Participants were subject to a wide variety of tests before, during and after the retreat using many measures, including biochemical, behavioral and electrophysiological. The overall goal was to ascertain the personal and physiological effects of intensive meditation training.

Telomerase, an enzyme that helps DNA strands to lengthen, was significantly elevated in meditators.

One of the elements of the biochemical research focused on telomeres and telomerase. Telomeres are DNA sequences at the ends of chromosomes, and telomerase is an enzyme that helps telomeres to grow. As we age, or if we have certain health conditions (such as inherited anemia or skin and lung diseases), telomeres tend to shorten. When telomeres become too short, cells can no longer multiply. Research shows that some cancers, osteoarthritis and osteoporosis, depression, diabetes, obesity and heart disease are all more likely to arise in people with shorter telomeres. So it is fair to say that longer telomeres equal longevity and in order to have longer telomeres one must have telomerase in one's system.

The research demonstrated that telomerase was significantly elevated in the meditators. Project researcher Elissa Epel, a psychologist from the University of California, San Francisco (UCSF), in collaboration with UCSF's Elizabeth Blackburn (who shared the 2009 Nobel Prize in Physiology or Medicine for her work on telomeres), discovered that telomerase levels were about one-third higher in the white blood cells of retreat participants compared to controls.

Saron states, "We have found that meditation promotes positive psychological changes and that meditators showing the greatest improvement on various psychological measures had the highest levels of telomerase. The effect appears to be attributable to psychological changes that increase a person's ability to cope with stress and maintain feelings of wellbeing."

The work on telomerase was just one small aspect of the Shamatha project, which has taken over eight years and cost more than $4 million. Other tests measured cognitive ability and emotional regulation.

When asked about his goal for this research, Saron expresses a profoundly compassionate perspective: "My hope is that individuals understand their interior life better and find ways to wrest a kind of vitality and creativity from their ongoing lived experience."

Saron's research correlates with other studies that have demonstrated physiological and psychological benefits of regular meditation practice. While his experiment involved intensive meditation practice for a minimum of six hours a day over a three-month period of residential retreat, other research has shown significant changes (not known to be related to telomerase) with short daily practice periods trained within a 10-week non-residential program.

For example, the Mindfulness Based Stress Reduction (MBSR) program, founded by Dr. Jon Kabat-Zinn and headquartered at the University of Massachusetts Medical School's Center for Mindfulness, has been used as a framework to study the effect of mindfulness meditation practice on chronic pain. In one study, 51 chronic pain patients who had not responded to conventional medical care showed significant reduction of pain (65 percent had a reduction of 33 percent and half showed a reduction of 50 percent). In another clinical trial, patients with moderate to severe psoriasis, who underwent ultraviolet light treatment while listening to guided meditation recordings, healed at approximately four times the rate of subjects receiving the light treatment alone.

Other research from the Center for Mindfulness correlates the practice of meditation with increased happiness. Renowned psychologist Daniel Goleman (the author of *Emotional Intelligence and The Brain* and *Emotional Intelligence: New Insights*) wrote in *The New York Times* about a collaborative research project between Kabat-Zinn and Dr. Richard Davidson, director of the Laboratory for Affective Neuroscience at the University of Wisconsin.

Just three hours per week of meditation training over eight weeks, elevated mood, increased energy and reduced anxiety.

Before the collaboration, Davidson had discovered that subjects with higher activation in the right prefrontal cortex were more inclined to be anxious and depressed, whereas those with positive, upbeat mood states had more activation in the left. The joint research found that stressed bio-tech workers shifted their frontal lobe orientation from right to left over the course of meditation training involving only three hours a week over eight weeks. As Goleman states, "…their moods improved, they reported feeling engaged again in their work, more energized and less anxious…Davidson hypothesizes that [meditation training] may strengthen an array of neurons in the left prefrontal cortex that inhibit the messages from the amygdala that drive disturbing emotions." This research also showed that workers who underwent the meditation training had stronger immune systems.

Hmmm…a potentially younger body, a happier mind and improved immune system? If a drug obtained these results in pre-market research, I suspect that millions of dollars would be invested in bringing it to market. Shareholders of the drug company discovering this fountain of vitality would be thrilled.

Elizabeth Blackburn and Elissa Epel, both mentioned earlier in this chapter with respect to telomerase, have already jumped on the commercial bandwagon as two of the co-founders of Telome Health Inc., a company that tests individuals' telomere length as a measure of health status and disease risk.

I wonder what intrinsic value such testing will bring to our lives? Several key determinants of health and longevity have been clearly established: having enough money for our basic needs, good nutrition, exercise and sufficient sleep. Many individuals are already investing in lengthening their telomeres through regular meditation practice. If governments started funding mindfulness meditation training programs, fewer people would need medical care. Some businesses are catching on and teaching mindfulness meditation in the workplace because they see the benefit of having healthier, happier and more engaged employees.

This is such good news, let's celebrate and shift more frontal lobes to the left!

*The brain is a wonderful
organ; it starts working the
moment you get up in the
morning and does not stop
until you get into the office.*

Robert Frost

Chapter 4

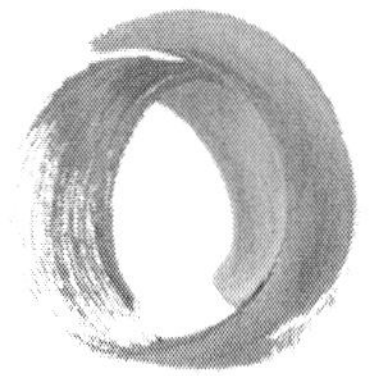

Back to the Cradle?
Rocking the Brain to Sleep

Scientists have confirmed what mothers have known for eons: you can get the best rest by dozing in a hammock or on another gently swinging surface.

A study by Swiss researchers showed that napping on a slowly swinging surface activates the parts of the brain involved in sleep. The swinging motion propelled healthy male subjects in the study more rapidly into sleep and gave them longer-lasting deep sleep than sleeping on a non-rocking surface.

Sophie Schwartz, the University of Geneva sleep scientist who led the study, said it confirms what mothers have long known intuitively when they rock their babies to sleep.

"The use of rocking to induce sleep thus belongs to our repertoire of adaptive behaviors in which a natural mechanism of sleep ... has been harnessed in the simplest manner since immemorial times," wrote Dr. Schwartz and her colleagues in the report of their findings, published on June 21, 2011 in the journal *Cell Biology*. To test their hypothesis that swinging can improve human sleep, Dr. Schwartz and her colleagues studied 12 healthy, male volunteers aged 22 to 38. They examined each subject's sleep parameters while he took an afternoon nap in a completely dark room on a custom-made bed that was stationary in one 45-minute test and rocking gently in another. All of the men were good sleepers, did not normally take naps, had low anxiety levels and no excessive daytime sleepiness.

During the test when the bed was rocking, the motion was sufficient to stimulate the subjects' vestibular sensory system – which keeps track of the body's movements – and the proprioceptive sensory system – which follows the relative positions of the parts of the body. It was not enough to cause nausea or variations in heart rhythms, however.

British billionaire Richard Branson is quoted in www.entrepreneur.com: I have the most beautiful office in the world – a hammock overlooking the British Virgin Islands! A fantastic place for reflection, it sets me up for the day and the surprises that are bound to happen. I come up with more ideas on that hammock than I ever would anywhere else.

Eight of the 12 men reported after the tests that sleeping while swinging was more pleasant than sleeping while remaining stationary; the others reported that both sleeping conditions were equally pleasant.

The research team found that rocking accelerated each participant's sleep onset. It also increased the duration of one stage of deep sleep and increased another parameter associated with restful or deep sleep known as spindle density.

In addition, rocking increased what the scientists described as the subjects' "EEG [electroencephalogram] power of slow-wave activity," particularly during the last third of one of the deepest stages of sleep. This refers to increased slow-wave activity in the brain, which is associated with the deepest form of sleep.

The scientists aren't sure why rocking has these effects. They think it may cause a synchrony of activity of neurons within the parts of the brain linked to sleep. Whatever the underlying mechanism, we can all sleep more soundly knowing that mothers know best.

It is good to rub and polish our brain against that of others.

Michel de Montaigne

Chapter 5

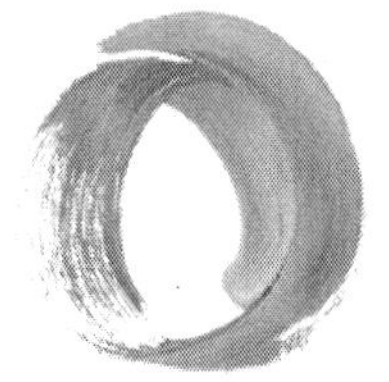

The Unsinkable Dr. Osborn

Sparkling intelligence, a happy home life and a high-powered career supervising medical interns in two hospital systems: Claudia Osborn, D.O., had it all. She wanted to be a doctor from the age of 10, and at 33, she was living her dream as a specialist in internal medicine.

That dream was shattered one sunny afternoon when she was struck by a car while cycling with her life partner, Marcia Baker. Osborn landed on her head, bringing her arms rigidly to her chest in a reflex typical of injury to the brain stem. She was drooling and unconscious. To Marcia, also a doctor, it must have been terrifying to witness Claudia in such obvious distress.

Over My Head is Osborn's account of living with a traumatic brain injury (TBI). The book takes readers along for a very bumpy ride, focusing chiefly on the 18 months of neurorehabilitation therapy Osborn received in New York City. It offers fascinating and often humorous insights into neurorehabilitation and the daily living challenges of someone with a TBI.

One of the things that amazed me was the fact that Osborn traveled from Detroit to New York alone and stayed in a series of friends' apartments for the first several months of her rehabilitation. Later, she lived alone in a one-room apartment. By the end of a full day of learning how to think and communicate again, she often went to bed hungry because she lacked the ability to plan to buy food or think about how to prepare it; she started a kitchen fire (which she was able to put out) by putting food on to cook but then forgot about it; threw her dirty laundry down the garbage chute; got lost countless times; and didn't know what to do when her phone stopped working.

Why on earth did her loved ones let her undertake this venture without greater support?

In an interview with BetterBrainBetterLife.com, Osborn says the answer is complex: "The simplest answer is ignorance. A damaged brain can't tell its owner that it's wounded or make good judgments. I wasn't used to people telling me what to do. I didn't believe I needed help. I agreed to go to New York for a few months (not the 20 it actually took) but only on my terms. When they learned of my failures, Marcia, my mother and two New York friends created safety nets. I still failed, but with less consequence. More importantly, while the daily challenges took a toll, they did foster my independence."

Osborn now realizes that she pushed herself too hard and that more support would have been in order. "I had some horrible experiences during that time," she admits.

In contrast to her uber-independence, many brain-injured people are over-protected by family and friends, says Osborn, who is now a consultant and lectures widely on brain injury rehabilitation to medical professionals and brain injury support groups.

"Brain-injured people need to be allowed to fail safely in order to realize that we can't do what we used to do without tailored strategies," she explains. "Too much direction lets us think we're coping. This makes it difficult to move out of the cocoon and work beyond our deficits. I tell my caregivers, walk behind me. If I'm lost let me figure it out. Just save me from being arrested for vagrancy on the public streets."

Many brain-injured people are over-protected by family and friends.

With the tragic death of Marcia, her partner of 25 years, Osborn had to learn more daily coping strategies. "I hate to admit that I only recently mastered the laundry. And I still have a coach who keeps me on track with administrative matters. But there hasn't been a year since the accident in 1978 that I haven't grown and changed. You may not notice much improvement from month to month, but over the course of a year a lot happens."

While Osborn wasn't able to recover the life she loved before the accident, she has created a life that is meaningful – and not only to her. She lectures in rehabilitation medicine throughout North America, and is an advisor on TBI education and prevention to several government agencies, including the Centers for Disease Control (CDC) in Atlanta, the National

Institutes of Health (NIH) in Washington DC, and the Michigan Department of Health.

Praised by *Publisher's Weekly*, *Over My Head* was an Alternate Selection of the Literary Guild Book Club, and a condensed book in the March, 1998 edition of *The Reader's Digest*. In the spring of 2001, *Psychology Today* honored Osborn for her contribution to mental health.

Osborn's book is funny, moving and above all inspiring. It moves along quickly until you suddenly feel like you have a new friend, someone you want to tell everyone about because she's conquered such tremendous odds and you feel so privileged to know her.

*Many highly intelligent people
are poor thinkers. Many people
of average intelligence are
skilled thinkers. The power
of a car is separate from the
way the car is driven.*

Edward de Bono

Chapter 6

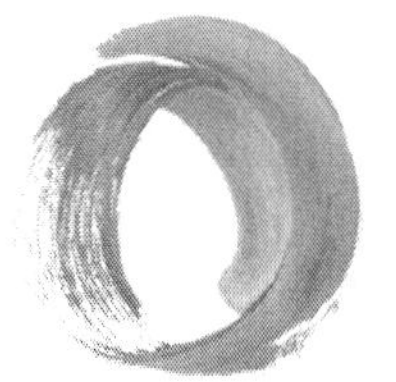

Grow Your Brain's Memory Center

There is now more tantalizing evidence that taking fish oil supplements can keep your brain supple for a longer time.

In a study presented at the 2011 International Conference on Alzheimer's disease in Paris, investigators showed that people who used fish oil supplements enjoyed better cognitive functioning over the course of the three-year study than those who didn't. They also had less reduction in brain volume over time. However, these associations only occurred among people with normal baseline cognitive function who did not carry the gene ApoE4, a known risk factor for Alzheimer's.

The team, from the Alzheimer's disease and Memory Disorders Center at the Rhode Island Hospital in Providence, RI, looked at data from the Alzheimer's disease Neuroimaging (ADNI) study. They focused on 819 people who had been recruited into the study between 2005 and 2010. Most had been taking fish oil supplements for at least the previous two years and took the supplements for at least six months after they entered the study. The ADNI study was a six-year multi-center initiative launched in 2004.

Researchers gathered information from a variety of sources, including cognitive testing and magnetic resonance imaging, in people who entered the study. The subjects included people without any cognitive impairment and those with mild cognitive impairment or Alzheimer's disease. Mild cognitive impairment is believed to occur before dementia sets in.

The study revealed that use of fish oil supplements was linked to better cognitive function, particularly as time went on. However, this was only true, in the final analysis, in those who did not carry the ApoE4 gene or who had normal cognitive function at baseline.

Intriguingly, the investigators also found that use of fish oil supplements is associated with higher volumes of some parts of the brain, including the cerebral cortex, which is where the higher cognitive functions are performed. But again, this was only true in those who did not carry the ApoE4 gene.

Even those with Alzheimer's showed an increase in the volume of brain regions involved in memory.

The researchers also examined the results according to whether the subjects had normal cognitive function at baseline, mild cognitive impairment or Alzheimer's. They found that members of all three groups had higher brain volumes over time, something that had never been found before. Even individuals with Alzheimer's experienced an increase in volume of the hippocampus, which is involved in short- and long-term memory.

"My personal bias is that supplementation of any type that might potentially delay cognitive decline or help prevent Alzheimer's disease probably needs to take place years before people would start to show symptoms," lead investigator Lori Daiello, PharmD, told BetterBrainBetterLife.com. "And the fact that we only saw positive effects in people who don't carry the ApoE4 gene suggests that people who do carry the gene may have more advanced changes in their brains at the time that they started taking the fish oil. So perhaps they would have had to start supplementation years earlier for it to have had an effect."

Daiello believes it would be useful to do longer-term studies of the effects of fish oil supplementation on cognitive decline.

I've got the brain of a four year old. I'll bet he was glad to be rid of it.

Groucho Marx

Chapter 7

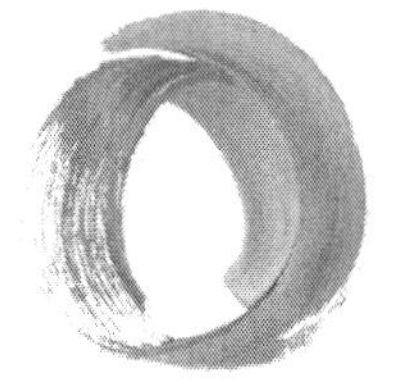

Does Your Heart Have a Brain?

Positive emotional experiences can indeed be a matter of choice, and practice, as Dr. Karen Shue, a neuropsychologist with a busy practice in Toronto knows.

Shue was trying to return home from a conference outside of New York. The airport was very small and all flights were temporarily grounded. She describes the scene: "The place was quickly filling up with hundreds of stranded passengers. It was hot, there were no seats and people were continually bumping into one another."

Knowing a thing or two about the power of the heart and its relationship to the brain, Shue, who received her Ph.D. in clinical psychology with a focus on neuropsychology from McGill University, started practicing heart coherence: focusing on the physical location of her heart, practicing deep, slow breathing and remembering a positive emotional experience from her past. Her mood and assessment of the situation improved and before long she noticed that the woman beside her was in a positive mood, too. They began to talk and laugh and before long they had attracted a group of other positive-minded individuals. "We were just hanging around, telling stories and laughing. We had such a good time that when the planes started to fly again we all hugged each other goodbye. Then, as a bonus, when my plane took off, I witnessed the most glorious sunset of my life."

Shue often uses a program called HeartMath® with her clients. "It helps you pay attention to what is working in your life and to investigate what you can appreciate in any situation. As an example, a client was having problems relating to people at work. Through HeartMath she learned to disengage from her judgments of co-workers and to be more open to their points of view. She was subsequently promoted. Her personal life improved tremendously, too: her boyfriend of several years proposed to her, noting that he was appreciating her 'softer side.' "

HeartMath is a leader in heart-brain research and offers programs and technologies for individuals and groups.

HeartMath exercises can be done with or without technology. The book, *The HeartMath Solution*, by Doc Childre and Howard Martin, gives instructions. You can also purchase biofeedback software that helps develop what is called heart coherence, or more appropriately, psycho-physiological coherence.

Coherence can be defined as integration and harmony among the components of a system. According to HeartMath research, when you focus on the heart center (the physical location of the heart in the chest), breathe deeply and rhythmically and recall positive emotions your heart, brain and autonomic nervous system begin to function in a more coherent way.

In an interview with BetterBrainBetterLife.com, Howard Martin said, "Brain function is critically dependent on signals coming from the heart. With every beat, the heart transmits complex patterns of neurological, hormonal, blood pressure and electromagnetic information to the brain and throughout the body."

The heart muscle is composed of neuronal proteins and support cells that communicate with the brain through neuropathways that originate in the heart and enter the brain through the medulla, pass through the limbic system and terminate in the neurocortex. Says Martin, "There are approximately 40,000 neurons in the heart and a large number are local circuit neurons, the same as those used for memory functions in the brain."

Heart Rate Variability (HRV) is a term used to describe a measure of the beat-to-beat changes in heart rate. These changes are influenced by emotions thoughts and physical exercise. Imagine looking at a graph of a beating heart. Typically we look only at the spikes that indicate a pulse. But what the graph shows between those pulses is very telling: clearly indicating, for example, the difference between a person who is angry and one who is calm. Optimizing one's HRV affects decision-making capacity, ability to solve problems and creativity.

Deep, regular breathing can serve to enhance HRV on its own but according to HeartMath research (much of which has been published in peer-reviewed scientific journals) such breathing, combined with focus on the heart and the evocation of positive emotions, results in optimal HRV (also referred to as a coherent heart). Benefits of the practice include a reduction in cortisol (the stress hormone) and an elevation in DHEA, an anti-aging, energizing, anti-stress adrenal hormone. In a 1998 study, just one month of HeartMath practice resulted in an average increase of 100 percent in the DHEA levels of subjects.

Karen Shue's airport experience may have been facilitated by her heart's electromagnetic field, which is 5,000 times greater than the field generated by the brain. The energy of a coherent heart can be measured as far as 15 feet from the body. HeartMath research showed that when two people touch, the electrical energy generated by one person's heart (as represented by the tracings on an EEG is detected in the brain of the other. So the crowded conditions in the airport may have facilitated the spread of positive emotions amongst those standing near Shue.

The electromagnetic field of the heart is 5,000 times stronger than that of the brain.

HeartMath's emwave® biofeedback software measures pulse and HRV and feeds real-time information to the user in the form of graphs, colored lights and games (depending on user selection). While you don't need the technology to practice heart coherence, it can enhance focus and motivation.

Generating positive emotional states has been shown in other research to enhance brain function. In the New York

Times bestselling book *RAPT: Attention and the Focused Life*, Winifred Gallagher, states:

> Not only how you focus, but also what you focus on can have important neurophysiological and behavioral consequences. Just as one-pointed concentration on a neutral target, such as your breath, particularly strengthens certain of the brain's attentional systems, meditation on a specific emotion – unconditional love – seems to tune up certain of its affective networks. In experiments, when monks who are focusing on this feeling of pure compassion are exposed to emotional sounds, brain activity increases in the insula, a region involved in visceral perception and empathy, and in the right temporo-parietal junction, an area implicated in inferring and empathizing with others' mental states. These data complement research done by Barbara Fredrickson and others showing that concentration on positive emotions improves your affect and expands your focus. Davidson speculates that deliberately focusing on feelings such as compassion, joy and gratitude may strengthen neurons in the left prefrontal cortex and inhibit disturbing messages from the fear-oriented amygdala.

Martin says that when we are in the coherent state, "we are more acutely aware of what we are thinking and feeling and more aware of other people and the environment. This greater degree of sensitivity allows for better discernment and improves our lives as spouses, parents and in the workplace."

Telling the story of the heart and how it communicates with the brain and the rest of the body has been

HeartMath's contribution to science, according to Martin. As the gospel of heart-focused personal change grows and awareness spins out from the personal to the family and on to the broader community, Martin sees HeartMath making a contribution to global consciousness.

The transition into heart intelligence will be more significant than the transition from the Middle Ages to the Renaissance and Scientific Revolution, or the transition from the Industrial Revolution to the Information Age of the past century. It represents a dimensional shift in human awareness – and it's already started.

*See, I think we have to
ask ourselves — and this is
corny in a way — what are we
doing here. And I've become
convinced, after a lifetime of
asking that question, that
we are here to enlarge our
souls, light up our brains,
and liberate our spirits.*

Tom Robbins

Chapter 8

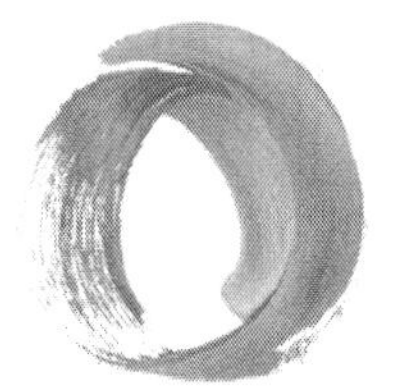

The Nature of the Brain?
Who Really Knows?

The world of science and the world of spirituality may be moving closer together, at least in the minds of many of us who find this prospect tantalizing. But Stephen Hawking, one of the great minds of our time, doesn't see it this way. I found this quote about the brain from Hawking, and later another by Nobel-laureate Sir John C. Eccles, which is diametrically opposed. I then asked Dallas, TX-based neuroscientist Dr. Gerald Kozlowski to read them and weigh in.

Quote One:

I regard the brain as a computer, which will stop working when its components fail. There is no heaven or afterlife for broken down computers; that is a fairy story for people afraid of the dark.

Stephen Hawking, interview in The Guardian
(May 15, 2011)

Quote Two:

I maintain that the human mystery is incredibly demeaned by scientific reductionism, with its claim in promissory materialism to account eventually for all of the spiritual world in terms of patterns of neuronal activity. This belief must be classed as a superstition…We have to recognize that we are spiritual beings with souls existing in a spiritual world as well as material beings with bodies and brains existing in a material world.

Sir John C. Eccles, Evolution of the Brain: Creation of the Self (1991)

Kozlowski Weighs In:

The contrast in philosophies between these two giant thinkers is deserving of examination, for they could hardly be more opposed.

I find it surprising that Stephen Hawking reduces the brain to the status of a machine, albeit a sophisticated one. He's not alone in likening the brain to a computer, but there are incredibly important distinctions that need to be made.

The brain is living and labile with plastic properties (i.e. the ability to change in response to experience), unlike the hard-wired, indeed soldered connections of a circuit board, which are incapable of change. In contrast to a computer, neuronal synapses respond to increased use and the strength of the synapse grows in power according to use. A much-used neuronal circuit can improve, which is the basis for improved performance that accompanies the practice of the musician or athlete.

Hawking states that the brain "will stop working when its components fail." While it is true that there are indeed traumatic events, diseases and disorders that can overwhelm the brain and lead to brain death, the brain, nevertheless, has the ability to repair itself in amazing ways, thought to be impossible a mere 20 years ago. There are numerous examples of the brain replacing lost function in response to training, and of one part of the brain automatically taking over for another when the first becomes dysfunctional. Stem cell and genetic medical research hold the promise for even greater miracles to occur in the future. These plastic properties make the brain entirely unlike a computer.

Another feature of the brain that Hawking downplays is the parallel distributive nature of brain circuitry. His quote, despite the fact it may be in a completely acceptable context, reveals his perception that the brain operates through serial (or linear) processing.

If the brain operated serially then, yes, the whole system would break down if there were an error in just one step of a process. Depending on the extent of the failure, it could, indeed, totally stop, as in brain death seen after stroke. Most of the time, however, the brain processes in a parallel fashion, i.e., it can process multiple bits of information simultaneous-ly, and in ways that are likely far more complex than we currently understand. In fact, unlike the soldered connection of a circuit motherboard, neuronal connections separate from and rejoin their targets (other neuronal cell bodies, muscles and glands) in a dynamic, multidimensional dance that make binary code (the zeros and ones of computer language) look positively Neanderthal. Even the development of artificial intelligence capabilities used by supercomputers pales in comparison to the complex functioning of the human brain.

There is one way in which the computer *is* superior to the brain: components in a computer can sometimes be replaced when a hard drive has crashed. We are certainly not at the point where this is possible with the brain. However, when a particular brain circuit fails, the brain can usually be trained, or will train itself, to compensate, albeit with some functional deficit remaining, as mentioned above.

Sir John's philosophy is much more realistic, given the oft-espoused belief that humans have both a material and immaterial nature. This is in alignment with the brain-body-spirit-connection thinking that is gaining credibility. According to this view, which I happen to share, the brain may be viewed as a sort of a funnel for consciousness, a means by which the infinitely broader transpersonal reality of consciousness is expressed in a human being.

*You have two hemispheres
in your brain — a left and a
right side. The left side controls
the right side of your body and
right controls the left half.
It's a fact. Therefore, left-
handers are the only people in
their right minds.*

Bill Lee
left-handed Major League pitcher
1969-1982

Chapter 9

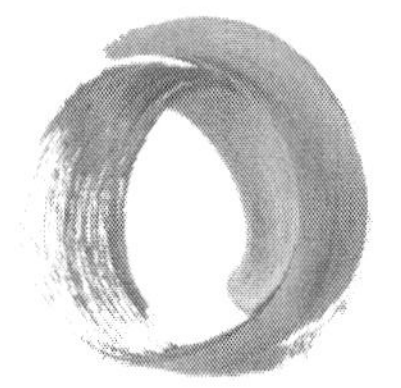

Food For Thought:
Does Soy Enhance Your Brain?

If you're 45+ you may well be searching for something (*anything*) that will help keep your mind and memory strong as you age. Could soy foods be helpful – or do they harm the brain as some research suggests?

A study from Stanford University, published in the June 2012 issue of *Neurology*, reveals the effects of soy on 313 postmenopausal women. Over the course of two and a half years, half of the participants were given a daily dose of soy equal to the amount found in a typical Asian diet; the other group was given a placebo. The women took memory and thinking ability tests at the beginning and end of the study, which found that while their overall cognition did not improve, there was a small but significant improvement (13 percent) in visual recognition, including the recognition of faces, in the group of women that took soy.

While the study's lead author Victor W. Henderson, MD, MS, concludes that adding soy to the diet neither harms nor benefits users, I'm guessing that a 13 percent improvement in facial recognition would be most welcome by anyone having trouble remembering faces. The ability to recognize faces is a key aspect of a good social life, and other research indicates that a good social life is a key component of remaining mentally young.

Those receiving soy showed improvements in episodic memory.

Dr. Sandra E. File, Ph.D. is a leading researcher in neuroscience and pharmacology, and the director of the Psychopharmacology Research Unit, Centre for Neuroscience, King's College, London. In an article published on www.soyconnection.com, File says that at least three reputable studies have demonstrated a positive correlation between soy supplementation and cognition. Two of those studies focus on postmenopausal women. File states that in one study, "Those receiving the soy supplement showed significantly greater improvements in episodic memory (e.g. immediate recall of a story or delayed recall of pictures) and in tasks measuring frontal lobe function (including the ability to plan)," while in another, "Those receiving the soy showed… greater improvements in story recall and in planning tasks."

In contrast, other research has shown soy products to have a negative effect on cognition over time. One of the best known studies was on Japanese-American men, between 1965–1967 and 1971–1974. While this study indicated reduced cognition among tofu eaters, it appears that the study was not controlled (for example, it relied on after-the-fact reports of how much tofu was eaten over a 20-year period) and its findings are therefore not reliable, according to File.

An article by Jack Norris, RD, from VeganHealth.org, points out that different types of soy products may produce different results, and that the way the food is prepared can have a significant effect. According to Norris, the poison formaldehyde was (and possibly still is) used in the preparation of tofu in Indonesia.

Norris says that soy is one of the most researched foods. He states, "Between 1990 and 2010 there were over 10,000 peer-reviewed journal articles on soy." Sorting the wheat from the chaff in all this research is no easy task and Norris points out that it is relatively easy for anyone to bolster an argument for or against soy by citing studies that may be less than reliable. Norris presents an excellent review of the research and should be read by those who want more information.

Norris' conclusion is that the jury is still out on the topic of soy and cognition. But he doesn't have concerns about adverse effects: "Based on the research to date, there should be little concern about eating soy, including tofu, with regards to cognitive decline."

The brain is wider than the sky;
For put them side by side
The one the other will contain
with ease — and you beside.

                                              Emily Dickinson

Chapter 10
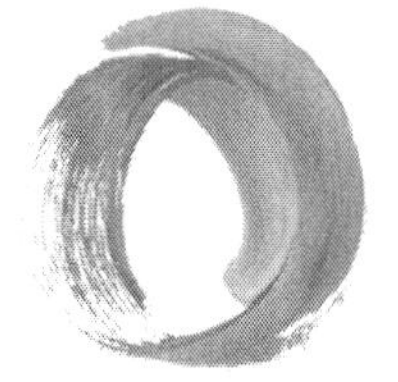

Seniors Lift Their Way to Brain Power

How many reps give you a better brain? Dr. Teresa Liu-Ambrose has a pretty good idea, and it's good news for seniors.

Liu-Ambrose has a long-standing interest in how exercise can improve the lives of older people. She recently found that seniors who engage in a regular program of resistance, or weight training, improve both their cognitive function and brain function.

"There is solid evidence that aerobic exercise relates to cognitive improvement and neuroplasticity. I wanted to look at strength training to see if it was equally beneficial," said Liu-Ambrose.

Originally trained as a physiotherapist, Liu-Ambrose is an Assistant Professor with the Department of Physical Therapy, University of British Columbia (UBC) and an investigator with both the Brain Research Centre and the Centre for Hip Health and Mobility in Vancouver. Her research focuses on aging, physical activity, mobility and cognitive health.

The Brain Power Study (published in *Archives of Internal Medicine*) undertaken by Liu-Ambrose followed 155 people, age 65–75. Some trained once a week and some twice a week, for a year. Both groups experienced benefits compared with the control group, who were doing a stretch and tone program. Interestingly, there was no significant difference in cognitive improvement between the once-a-week and twice-a-week groups. The degree of cognitive improvement was 11–13 percent.

Is this gain significant? Can an 11–13 percent improvement in cognition make a difference in a person's daily life? When asked this question, Liu-Ambrose said that program participants certainly felt that it did. In a sub-study, program participants received disposable cameras and were asked to take photos that might describe what it meant to them to be in the program. They were also asked to put captions on the photos. Responses were positive, with participants indicating that they were engaging with others more often and spending more time with family. One participant took a photo of a bull's eye on a curling rink with the caption, "Not quite out of the game yet."

A one-year follow-up study, again published in the *Archives of Internal Medicine* showed startling results. "We were very surprised to discover that the group that sustained cognitive benefits was the once-weekly strength training group rather than the twice-weekly training group," says Liu-Ambrose. "What we realized was that this group was more successful at being able to maintain the same level of physical activity achieved in the original study."

In fact, those in the twice-weekly group experienced a decline in fitness status compared to when they began the original study, while the once-weekly strength training group and the control group were able to maintain the higher levels of activity they achieved.

Liu-Ambrose's goal is to influence public policies that lead to practical life changes for seniors and she hopes this work on strength training and cognition will be influential. "The more evidence we have that exercise makes a difference the more likely we are to find uptake, not just by individual consumers but also with respect to government policies," she explains. "Perhaps seniors can obtain financial benefits from governments for participating in exercise programs just as people with children sometimes do. And treatment programs may start to implement weight training for people with, or at risk for dementia."

The group that did the strength training used fewer health resources.

The follow-up study also proved there was an economic benefit to once-weekly strength training. Health economists Jennifer Davis and Carlo Marra, research scientists with UBC's Faculty of Medicine, demonstrated that up to 12 months after the end of the Brain Power Study, this group used fewer health resources and had fewer falls than the twice-weekly group and the control group.

"This suggests that once-weekly resistance training is cost-saving, and the right type of exercise for seniors to achieve maximum economic and health benefits," says Davis.

The potential payback could be significant, given that cognitive decline is a key risk factor for falls. According to the Public Health Agency of Canada, data shows that "almost 62 percent of injury-related hospitalizations for seniors are the result of falls." And reducing falls, as a matter of public policy would save money: "A reduction in falls by 20 percent could result in an estimated 7,500 fewer hospitalizations and 1,800 fewer permanently disabled seniors; some $138 million annually could be saved nationally."

> *Cognitive decline is a key risk factor for falls.*

Thanks to the work of Dr. Liu-Ambrose, we now know that brain health and weight training can contribute to brain-healthy senior citizens. Let's hope governments around the world see the many advantages of making it easy for senior citizens to become and stay active. Tax incentives and easy access to facilities, along with trainers, would make a huge difference in healthy aging.

*If the brain were so simple
that we could understand it,
we would be so simple that
we couldn't.*

*Attributed to George E. Pugh in
The Biological Origins of
Human Values*

Chapter 11

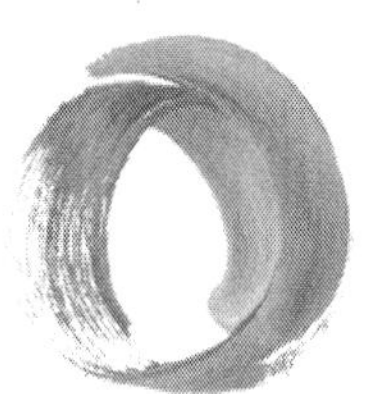

Brain Games for Self-Esteem

Brain games can be fun (when they're not too overwhelming) and MindHabits is an excellent example of brain games with proven positive benefits. MindHabits offers four games designed to train attention away from negative social and environmental inputs and towards positive ones. I played the trial version a few times, many days apart, and each time I found it enhanced my outlook.

Dr. Mark Baldwin is one of the inventors of the games, and the President and Chief Scientific Officer of MindHabits, a Montreal–based company. He also teaches psychology at McGill University.

"Our starting point is research showing that feelings of insecurity and daily stress arise in large part from anxieties about whether one will be liked, accepted and respected by one's peers and significant others," notes Baldwin. "Many people are oriented toward stress by noticing perceived social threats like rejection. This happens in a split second, below the radar of consciousness."

When I told Dr. Baldwin that playing the games enhances my mood, he said they don't typically find a straightforward mood effect in lab tests. "There may be something about the online game that is more fun than the version we do in the lab," he explains. "We tend to look for the effects on the way people process information."

Mental habits built up over years can make the world seem unfriendly and threatening.

Mental habits arise from the manner in which the brain processes information. They include being on the lookout for social threats like criticism or rejection, and are learned from our earliest interactions with others. Over time and with experience, we develop deep layers of unconscious thoughts and feelings about ourselves and the world around us, which make the world appear to be a more (or less) threatening place. Our level of self-esteem, sense of safety in social interactions, and the ability to form trusting relationships affect us in subtle and not-so-subtle ways. Life can be difficult when self-esteem is low.

The good news is that the degree to which individuals respond to negativity can be precisely measured via testing, and can be changed by playing these games. As Baldwin explains: "We have found via scientific testing that we can train the brain to disengage from negative social threats and negative thoughts about the self. At the same time our games direct the players' awareness toward positive experiences and thought-patterns."

The games were tested in the high-stress work environment of a call center, where employees are subject to constant rejection. The employees played the games every morning. "We measured their stress levels and confidence daily and their cortisol levels (a stress-response hormone) at the end of the week. Playing the games had a lasting effect under those conditions," notes Baldwin. "Interestingly, their sales went up as well."

Students are less aggressive after playing MindHabits.

In another test, high school students took occasional breaks to play the games and reported feeling less stressed about exams. And children aged 12–15 experienced a reduction in aggressive feelings after playing the games.

MindHabits staff continually tweak the programs, upgrading the games for new platforms and exploring other applications for the concept of improving self-esteem and mental health through games. "Collaborators are in the early stages of research on using the games for depression and eating disorders," says Baldwin.

MindHabits is careful to position itself as a non-therapeutic, fun product that is based on science.

As for me, I'm going to purchase the program for home use. At $19.95, what do I have to lose, except some negative programming?

*I like nonsense, it wakes up
the brain cells. Fantasy is a
necessary ingredient in living;
it's a way of looking at life
through the wrong end of a
telescope. Which is what I do,
and that enables you to laugh
at life's realities.*

Dr. Seuss

Chapter 12

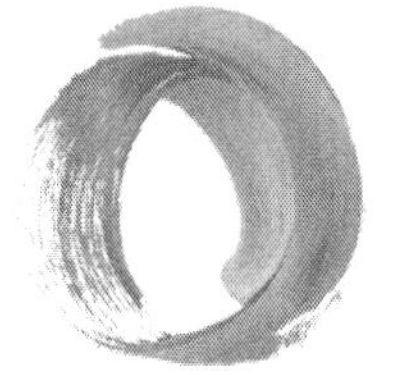

Wake Up and Smell the Cortex:
Our Senses Spark Brain Health

There's no doubt that evocative scents – a linden tree in bloom, a long-lost lover's perfume – have the power to evoke memories of the past and provoke feelings we thought long dead. How does this happen?

According to Manning Rubin, co-author with the late Lawrence Katz of *Keep Your Brain Alive*, memory is enhanced when more than one sense is involved in an experience; if you *touch* a rose, *smell* it and have strong *emotions* toward the person who handed it to you, your cortex is activated in at least three areas, creating a pattern and increasing the linkage between the cortical areas.

"Most of what we learn and remember relies on the ability of the brain to form and retrieve associations in much the same way Pavlov's dogs learned that the sound of a bell meant food," notes Rubin, a former advertising creative director who became interested in the field of brain science when he learned that adult brains are able to grow new cells. Rubin reasoned that there might be brain exercises that could help to stimulate such growth.

After meeting Lawrence Katz, a professor of neurobiology at Duke University Medical Center, the two men developed a systematic approach to exercising the brain for improved memory and overall mental flexibility. Their system, known as Neurobics, remains relevant today, 11 years after the first publication of their book, which has since been translated into 24 languages.

"Katz was a brilliant scientist and ahead of his time," notes Rubin. "He was working on growing dendrites (the branches on nerve cells that receive information from other cells) in rat brains and found that adding extra neurotrophins (a family of substances that induce the survival, development and function of neurons) to neurons almost doubles the size and complexity of the dendrites. It is actually the thinning out of dendrites that contributes to mental decline, so doubling the growth added a lot more mental horsepower."

It is now an accepted fact that while certain areas of the brain are "responsible" for specific sensory functions, the disuse of those functions can lead to cell atrophy and the possible appropriation of the area by another sensory function that is used to excess. This accounts for the heightened sense of touch in someone who uses her fingers to decipher Braille. In cases where a particular sensory area of the brain is not used, the senses become dull and presumably, life is less pleasurable. Those who no longer wake up and smell the coffee have lost the sense of excitement and wonder that a child is born with.

Rubin points out that most of us rely disproportionally on vision and hearing, neglecting the senses of touch, smell and taste. For instance, purchasing canned and frozen food in a grocery store prevents us from using our senses of touch and smell to determine the quality of the food. In contrast, shopping at a farmer's market engages more senses. And while text messaging uses touch when the fingers tap on a keyboard, we seldom use touch alone as a method of determining what something is, such as when we use our fingers with closed eyes to help us tell the difference between fur and leather.

Neurobics challenges us to combine our sensory experiences in new ways, and to break our routines and experience novel activities. The authors claim this will not only enhance mental fitness but help to seed new cell growth in the brain.

You'll recall that Lawrence Katz was experimenting with neurotrophins, substances that cause neurons to sprout new dendrites. *Keep Your Brain Alive* cites research demonstrating that neurotrophins help strengthen connections in the hippocampus, a part of the brain that is critical for learning and memory; the book also states that there is a direct correlation between nerve cell activity and the production of neurotrophins. So the more active a brain is, the more active it can become through the production of neurotrophins. Rubin likens this to a self-fertilizing garden: "Non-routine experiences that produce novel activity patterns in nerve cell circuits can produce greater quantities of neurotrophins."

These discoveries open up new opportunities for brain enhancement that are simple and accessible to all. What could be simpler than using the senses in novel combinations? Just as climbing the stairs is a physical exercise requiring no special equipment, Neurobics offers a simple way to exercise the brain in virtually any environment. In fact, Rubin and Katz have made it easy by offering 83 brain exercises for use in the workplace, while commuting, on arising or preparing for bed. As Rubin explains, "It's not about tricks, or about coming up with a few things that will help you remember a list of names – it's about how to live a life that is brain-healthy."

Neurobic Exercise Examples

- Introduce new scents and touch sensations to love-making.

- Find your clothes and get dressed with your eyes closed.

- Move familiar objects on your desk to new locations.

- Share a meal in silence.

- Eat with a blindfold on.

- Brush your teeth with your non-dominant hand.

- Keep a variety of scents at your desk and smell them when engaged in routine activities.

*Humor is by far the most
significant activity of the
human brain.*

Edward de Bono

Chapter 13

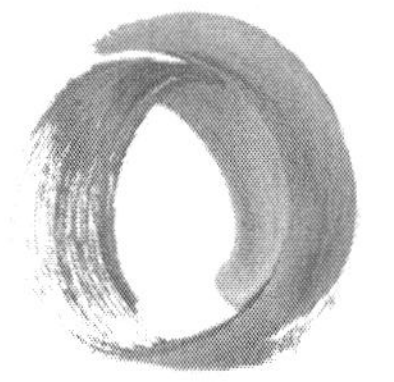

Watching the Adult Brain Grow: Eight Weeks to More Grey Matter

How can watching your mind change your brain? The concept of brain plasticity was given a concrete boost in 2005 when Harvard-based researcher Sara Lazar discovered thicker brain regions in people who practice mindfulness meditation. As far as we know, this was the first time anyone demonstrated that regular practice of a specific mental exercise can increase brain mass. The media enthusiastically applauded the news, and Lazar was interviewed for, or received mention in prestigious media outlets, including *National Geographic News*, *Time* and *The New York Times*.

A visit to Sara Lazar's website shows her impeccable academic credentials. She is an instructor in psychology at Harvard Medical School and a professor of psychiatry at Massachusetts General Hospital, where she specializes in functional magnetic resonance imaging (fMRI)). Lazar also has the ability to take life lightly, her humor coming through in some of the articles *(Search for Self Called Off)* and links to yoga videos for "you and your cat" on her site.

In an interview with BetterBrainBetterLife.com, Lazar described her research and talked about her life, motivations and her interest in building a bridge between science and the ancient practice of meditation.

First, the 2005 study: Lazar and her team started with the fact that the regular practice of meditation produces changes in mental states and electroencephalogram (EEG) patterns that last beyond the period of active practice. "We wondered if meditation practice might also result in significant cortical structural changes in regions that are engaged during the practice," she explains. "To test this hypothesis, we used magnetic resonance imaging to look at differences in the thickness of the cerebral cortex of experienced Buddhist Insight meditation practitioners."

Meditation offsets age-related cortical thinning.

Lazar defines Insight meditation thus: "The main focus is the cultivation of attention and a mental capacity termed "mindfulness," which is specific non-judgmental awareness of present-moment stimuli without cognitive elaboration. Formal practice involves sustained mindful attention to internal and external sensory stimuli."

Lazar and her research team were looking to see if there were differences in cortical thickness between meditators and non-meditators and also whether meditators with more experience would have greater thickness than those with less experience.

Twenty meditators, with between seven and nine years of experience, who practiced from four to six hours per week were matched with a control group of 15 non-meditators. The meditators had also participated in at least one weeklong retreat during which they practiced meditation for up to 10 hours per day. Participants were matched for sex, age, race and years of education.

Using magnetic resonance imaging, Lazar found increased cortical thickness in brain regions associated with attention, interoception (awareness of sensations inside the body) and sensory processing in the meditators. Thicker areas included the prefrontal cortex and right anterior insula. The research summary states, "Between-group differences in prefrontal cortical thickness were most pronounced in older participants, suggesting that meditation might offset age-related cortical thinning." In fact, in one brain region the average cortical thickness of the 40–50-year-old meditation participants was similar to the average thickness of the 20–30 year-old meditators and controls.

Two subsequent studies shed additional light on the relationship between meditation and grey matter growth and/or density. One, published in 2009, demonstrated reduced grey-matter density in the amygdala (known to play a role in anxiety and stress) in stressed but otherwise healthy individuals as a result of taking an eight-week course in mindfulness meditation. The second study, published in 2011, confirmed the previous finding on the amygdala and also discovered new areas of brain growth associated with participation in the same eight-week meditation program.

The Harvard news release states: "The analysis of MR images found increased grey-matter density in the hippocampus, known to be important for learning and memory, and in structures associated with self-awareness, compassion and introspection.

"Although no change was seen in a self-awareness-associated structure called the insula, which had been identified in earlier studies, the authors suggest that longer-term meditation practice might be needed to produce changes in that area. None of these changes were seen in the control group, indicating that they had not resulted merely from the passage of time."

Lazar's findings are consistent with a fundamental tenet of brain plasticity research: brain areas that are used repeatedly are strengthened. For example, repeated concentration on specific tasks like juggling or playing a musical instrument strengthens synaptic connections and sometimes increases the synaptic "real estate" of the regions of the brain "responsible" for those activities. It is unlikely that the observed differences in brain mass were due to pre-existing or incidental between-group differences (such as, for example, the possibility that the meditators were drawn to meditation practice because they already had greater brain mass).

What Led to this Research?

I couldn't help but wonder what led Sara Lazar to research the effect of meditation on cortical growth. As it turns out, it was the indirect result of injuries she sustained while running when she was a graduate student.

"I was a runner with knee and back problems and my physiotherapist said, 'Stop running and stretch.' On my way out of the office I saw a poster for a yoga class and decided to try it. After a while, I realized it was useful for stress reduction. At the end of each class there was a brief meditation period and I liked that. So I started to sit once a week and then more often. I've been meditating since 1997 and now practice four to five times a week."

Initially, Lazar was skeptical about some of the claims made for yoga and meditation. "Teachers make many unsubstantiated health claims and I wondered if there was any truth to them. Some of the existing research lacks credence, while some of it is verifiable. I was casting about for a research field and saw that the National Institutes of Health (NIH) were starting to fund research on alternative medicine. When I realized there was some serious scientific interest in things like yoga and meditation I didn't want to be left out."

Lazar turned a critical eye to some claims about yoga and meditation.

As for yoga research, Lazar has done a revised version of the 2005 study, this time comparing meditators and experienced yogis with one another and a control group. This work included research on how yoga itself affects the brain by studying before and after effects. The results are not yet published. Interestingly, despite creating such an impression in 2005, Lazar says it is still very difficult to get her work published.

Understandably, she won't discuss the study results before they are published in a peer-reviewed journal. "Back in the 1960s and 1970s there was so much bad research, and researchers would go public in yoga magazines and the like but nothing useful came out of it. At least with scientific journals you know there is a level of rigor applied to reviewing the research before it is published."

How do her academic colleagues receive her work? "It's mixed," she notes. "Some are completely skeptical and always will be and others are open to it. Most would agree that meditation has been proven useful for stress reduction. After all, it was 30 years ago that Jon Kabat-Zinn demonstrated with pre-and-post brain imaging that an eight-week course in mindfulness shrinks the amygdala and that this correlates with a reduction in stress."

A Spiritual Path?

Is the practice of meditation part of a spiritual path for Lazar?

"Meditation certainly changed my life in many ways. I'm not sure how much I want to say beyond that because people sometimes misconstrue what I say.

"One of the best ways to talk about the benefits of meditation in my life is that it is really good for helping me gain perspective in both my personal and work life. It helps me see things from multiple points of view and I'm better able to see solutions that incorporate those multiple viewpoints. It helps inform my research because I understand pretty clearly what we're aiming for, what will work and what won't. You might say that the world is less 'black and white' for me than it used to be and I handle stress much better."

Careful with her words, Lazar allows that she is, "not religious, but I am very interested in Buddhism and follow some of its guidelines." I ask if she considers herself a Buddhist. "I'm not sure. Most people who practice meditation in the U.S. don't call themselves Buddhist because of the religious beliefs that might be attributed to that term. Labeling my experience in that way is not useful."

Lazar finds no disconnect between science and meditation.

Lazar finds no disconnect between science and meditation. "Science is a search for the truth and Insight meditation is also about searching for truth. I am not researching enlightenment or esoteric states of consciousness but rather the bio-effects of the practice. As scientists, we know from 30 years of research that meditation reduces stress. How does that happen? That's what I'm trying to answer."

I had one last question, and it made her laugh, although perhaps ruefully. "Is the world of science as open to new ideas as you might like or expect?"

"Some of it is," she chuckles. "It's highly variable and some scientists are close-minded. Perhaps the fact that it's taking so long to have my work published is a reflection of those attitudes. It never seems to get easier but we'll see."

In the meantime, you can find Sara Lazar seeking truth, on the meditation cushion *and* in the lab.

It's called a pen. It's like a printer, hooked straight to my brain.

Dale Dauten

Chapter 14

A USB Port to the Brain

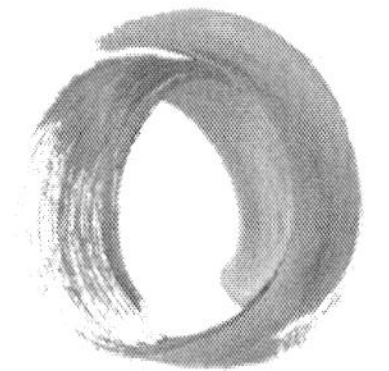

Stimulating your brain to change just became a lot easier, thanks to a new device that works its magic while you sleep.

This simple, drug-free, non-invasive device stimulates the nerves in the forehead with a mild electric current. The therapy, known as eTNS (external trigeminal nerve stimulation) stimulates the trigeminal nerve, which branches to the forehead, cheeks and jaw on both sides of the face. The electrical stimulation leads to cascading effects in the brain, including increased blood flow to, and hence improved function in, regions involved in depression, epilepsy and attention deficit hyperactivity disorder (ADHD).

The device is known as the Monarch eTNS system and is about the size of a cell phone. A wire is attached to a small patch that adheres to the user's forehead, over the trigeminal nerve, just above the eyebrows. The electrodes are attached to a pulse generator powered by a 9-volt battery (only a small fraction of the battery power is used to stimulate the nerves). The Monarch is typically worn during sleep, for between 8 and 12 hours, depending on the condition being treated.

The eTNS technology has been licensed to NeuroSigma, a Los Angeles-based medical device company. Dr. Ian Cook is director of Depression Research at UCLA and a scientific advisor to NeuroSigma. In an interview with BetterBrainBetterLife.com, Cook explained that even brief exposure to eTNS results in significant increases in cerebral blood flow in the anterior cingulate and the dorsomedial frontal cortical regions of the brain. These areas are implicated in mood disturbances.

Even brief exposure to the mild electrical current in this device increases cerebral blood flow.

"People with depression tend to have abnormally low levels of activity in that part of the brain," says Cook. "The signal we are sending via the trigeminal nerve is leading to changes in the firing of cells and part of the cascade of events is the increase in blood flow."

According to Cook, clinical improvements in depression are typically seen a week or two after the start of treatment. "This is still much better than medication for depression, which typically takes four weeks or longer to show results," he points out. "The idea of something entirely different, a 21st-century type of treatment, is very appealing; eTNS provides a high-bandwidth pathway to structures deep in the brain without the current penetrating directly through the skull."

A Phase II double-blind study of eTNS for the treatment of depression is under way.

The effect of eTNS on drug-resistant epilepsy is impressive. Two studies led by Dr. Christopher DeGiorgio of UCLA, who invented the eTNS device, showed that over 40 percent of patients using the system reported a 50 percent or better reduction in the number of seizures after 18 weeks of treatment. The research was published in the Journal Neurology in 2009 and 2013.

Forty percent of subjects with epilepsy achieved a 50 percent or greater improvement in seizure control.

People with epilepsy have few non-drug treatment options and many find that their condition is drug-resistant. Drugs may also have side effects. There is a surgical option of cranial nerve stimulation via the vagus nerve but that treatment involves hospitalization; eTNS must be welcome news indeed for those with epilepsy, a condition which can make a normal life next to impossible.

ADHD also responded well to eTNS in a study led by James McGough, Professor of Clinical Psychiatry at the Semel Institute for Neuroscience and Human Behavior and David Geffen School of Medicine at UCLA. In a Phase 1 study, improvements of over 45 percent after eight weeks of treatment were found in 20 subjects, aged seven to 14. Who knows – soon parents of children with ADHD might simply put their children to bed with the Monarch device and enjoy a blessedly relaxed and focused child the next day.

The Monarch eTNS device is currently approved for treatment of major depression and drug-resistant epilepsy in Canada and the European Union. Patients ages nine and older need a doctor's prescription to obtain it.

Cook notes that TNS offers several advantages over other treatments for both depression and epilepsy, including the fact that patients can administer it at home. "It is very cost-effective and quite competitive in terms of effectiveness when compared to invasive treatments," he says.

There is a foolish corner
in the brain of the wisest man.

Aristotle

Chapter 15

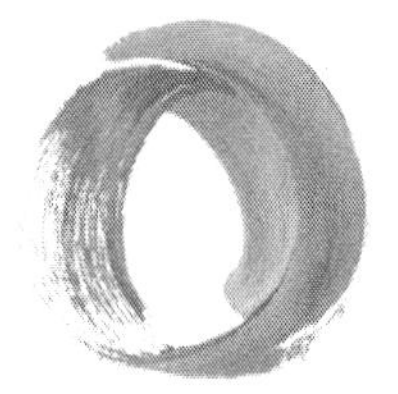

Can Eating Wheat
Make You Crazy, Lazy and Stupid?

The brain on gluten can be a frightening thing, and *Wheat Belly* is a "must read" if you've ever experienced the deplorable condition known as "brain fog" or if you're concerned about gluten in your diet.

But it doesn't stop there: if you have diabetes or celiac disease this book could save your mind or even your life. Likewise, if you or someone you care about has arthritis, digestive problems, even schizophrenia, you'll want to know about the possible implications of eating wheat.

BetterBrainBetterLife.com interviewed *Wheat Belly* author, cardiologist Dr. William Davis from his office in Milwaukee, WI. This chapter focuses on Davis' observations about the relationship between wheat and brain function.

But first some background.

It was the fact that 80 percent of his patients are either diabetic or pre-diabetic that got Davis wondering how their diet might be affecting their health. "It was a pretty simple conclusion," he explains. "I learned about the glycemic index, and realized that two slices of whole wheat bread increase blood sugar as much or more than table sugar or even many candy bars. So when I was devising a strategy to help my patients reduce blood sugar more efficiently, I could see that the quickest and simplest way to get results would be to eliminate wheat. I gave them a handout explaining how to replace wheat-based foods with other low-glycemic whole foods to create a healthy diet."

The results were astounding, says Davis. "Patients came back with incredible stories: 'I lost 30 pounds,' 'my arthritis is dramatically improved,' 'I've been able to stop taking acid reflux medicine,' 'my gas and cramps and diarrhea have stopped,' 'I don't need half the medication I was on before,' and so on."

Eating wheat spikes blood sugar, which can lead to fatigue and brain fog.

Initially, Davis attributed many of the reported benefits to coincidence: "How could ulcerative colitis go away just because the patient stopped eating wheat? But the link became very persuasive of causation when increasing numbers of patients reported similar wide-ranging benefits. And they would test it out by going off wheat and then on again, finding that their symptoms disappeared and then returned."

According to Davis' well-referenced book, the brain is influenced by wheat in several ways. One is the effect of the gliadin protein, a component of gluten. "The digestive by-products of gliadin protein are probably responsible for the addictive relationship many people have with wheat," notes Davis.

Wheat, addictive? Most definitely, says Davis. "Digestion of wheat yields exorphins, morphine-like compounds that bind to the brain's opiate receptors. Exorphins induce a mild euphoria. When the effect is blocked or when no exorphin-yielding foods are consumed, some people experience a distinctly unpleasant withdrawal."

Interestingly, wheat-eating people consume substantially fewer calories of any type of food, and significantly fewer wheat-based products when given opiate-blocking drugs. Davis says that drug companies are researching this relationship, presumably eager to sell weight loss drugs rather than have people remove addictive foods from their diets.

> *Morphine-like compounds in wheat bind to the brain's opiate receptors.*

The work of the late F. Curtis Dohan, an endocrinologist based in Philadelphia, was essential to the discovery of the wheat-brain connection. Dohan scoured then-extant research and found a connection between wheat consumption and schizophrenia in various populations, including hunter-gatherer societies in New Guinea, where, before the introduction of wheat, schizophrenia was virtually unknown. After grain was introduced to their diet this population saw the incidence increase from two out of 65,000 to numbers typical of western grain-consuming populations: one in 100.

Dohan also researched the effects of a wheat-free, milk-free diet on veterans admitted to the locked ward of the Veteran's Administration Hospital in Coatesville, PA, in the late 1960s. He found that patients on the controlled diet were released into open wards roughly twice as fast as those on a conventional diet. When gluten was secretly reintroduced to the diet of those patients, the fast release to open wards did not occur. In a later study, Dohan also found that schizophrenics who were on the restricted diet when living in locked wards were also released from the open wards sooner than those who had been on a conventional diet while in locked wards.

The incidence of schizophrenia appears to rise as populations consume more wheat.

Some effects of wheat consumption are easily reversible (as in the diverse symptoms mentioned above). But Davis claims that wheat may also contribute to irreversible brain damage.

Cerebellar ataxia (CA) is a sign of an underlying condition in which brain cells in the cerebellum become diseased or injured. CA, which affects physical coordination and balance, speech, eye movement and the ability to swallow, can be caused by alcoholism, stroke, cerebral palsy and many other conditions. Davis posits a connection between CA and wheat consumption, referring to studies that show abnormal blood markers for gluten in 50 percent of those afflicted with ataxia for which no other cause can be identified, and in 20 percent of people with all forms of ataxia.

Furthermore, 10 to 22.5 percent of people with celiac disease are at risk of developing nervous system problems, such as cerebellar ataxia, which may also cause impaired memory and verbal abilities.

In his telling of the CA/wheat story Davis appears to overstate the facts. The description of CA and the lack of any background information on the condition led me on first reading to assume that the condition has no other causes than wheat consumption and that it is always fatal. Further research reveals a variety of causes, as mentioned above, as well as the fact that CA is most common in young children, following a viral infection such as chicken pox. The National Institutes of Health website states that while permanent symptoms are possible, "People whose condition was caused by a recent viral infection should make a full recovery without treatment in a few months."

Unfortunately, hyperbole, such as the statement that the horrible death likely from CA is "due to the muffins and bagels you so crave," weakens Davis' book. However, the fact that wheat consumption can lead to this dreadful condition is certainly worth publicizing. And, after reading an early version of this chapter, Davis responded:

> Overstated? Hmmm. While perhaps I am guilty of overstating the role of wheat exposure in causation of cerebellar ataxia and other degenerative neurologic conditions, how many other causes, 1) can be cured with elimination of a food, and are 2) curable without drugs, devices, or other elaborate maneuvers?
>
> Truly, the enormity of this nutritional blunder is hard to overstate. Just the mere fact that many people

from the drug industry are actually principals in the grain lobby alone should be reason to ask why this awful situation has been allowed to occur.

Surely there is more to brain health and optimal brain functioning than elimination of wheat. I too, am fascinated by all the various facets of brain and mind health, having toyed with such things as piracetam and ergoloid mesylates. But what if the collective IQ and level of functioning of a nation were to be boosted even five percent by a simple shift in diet?

Gluten encephalopathy is a brain disease that shows symptoms similar to those of cerebellar ataxia. Davis recounts, "one particularly disturbing Mayo Clinic study of 13 patients with the recent diagnosis of celiac disease in which dementia was also diagnosed. Of those 13, frontal lobe biopsy or postmortem examination of the brain failed to identify any other pathology beyond that associated with wheat gluten exposure. Of the 13, nine died due to progressive impairment of brain function."

Dr. Davis struggled to maintain focus as his blood sugar levels soared.

As mentioned earlier, eating wheat spikes blood sugar, typically leading to a burst of energy followed by a precipitous decline in blood sugar that leaves one feeling enervated. Lack of mental clarity is a result.

This is where brain fog comes in. Dr. Davis was no stranger to brain fog himself. "I struggled with brain fog and overwhelming sleepiness during the day for over 20 years," he explains. "I would eat whole grains, drink coffee and constantly struggle to maintain focus and attention. I was shocked to realize that my blood sugar levels were in the diabetic range even though I supposedly ate well and exercised almost every day. I have none of those problems now. I can go on three hours of sleep and feel fine."

The fatigue caused by eating wheat can be more than just a blood sugar effect, notes Davis. "For me, it can take 36 to 48 hours for the effect of two slices of bread to wear off. That is well beyond the time needed for blood sugar to stabilize. I don't know why that is. When one begins looking at the effects of wheat there are a lot more questions than answers."

Davis is eager to see more research conducted into the relationship between wheat consumption and health. As he has observed, both personally and professionally, "The tangle of health consequences associated with wheat consumption is truly impressive."

Davis has written an excellent book that raises important questions. Individuals who choose to follow his advice have little to lose (except some excess weight) and stand to gain in terms of mental and physical health. While this chapter has focused on the wheat-brain connection *Wheat Belly* is much more comprehensive in its discussion of a wide range of health issues, including diabetes, irritable bowel, celiac disease, arthritis, dermatology and aging.

Dr. Peter H. Dohan, a Cape Breton, NS-based surgical pathologist and the son of aforementioned pioneering researcher Dr. F. Curtis Dohan, is a big fan of *Wheat Belly*, despite the fact that Davis wrongly states that F.C. Dohan was a psychiatrist (he was an endocrinologist).

"I am a very well-informed physician and I read the book four times," says Dohan. "I keep reading it because every time I learn something new. It reads like a medical textbook in many ways, providing a lot of information to the general public that isn't well known. It is a marvelous book."

*Try not thinking of peeling an
orange. Try not imagining the
juice running down your
fingers, the soft inner part of
the peel. The smell. Try and
you can't. The brain doesn't
process negatives.*

Doug Coupland

Chapter 16

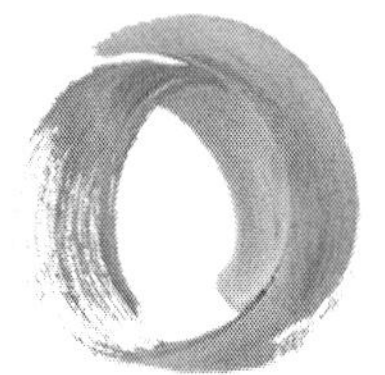

Students Free Up Brain Power

Do I belong? Am I good enough? Am I safe? Am I smart enough? Most of us are familiar with the anxieties that affect students of all ages.

Questions like those above are emotional in nature and while they are more or less "natural," if they loom too large they can negatively impact success by impeding the brain's processing power.

Recent research speaks to the emotional needs of students and their relationship to success. The first study uses expressive writing, the second teaches meditation and the third involves students in a program that gives them insight into issues of belonging. Each course of action helps to free up brainpower, allowing students to succeed both socially and academically.

Strategy Number One: Expressive Writing

Researchers at the University of Chicago (UChicago) wanted to know if students with test anxiety would benefit from expressive writing about their fears.

"We reasoned that if worries lead to poor test performance, and writing helps regulate these worries, then giving students the opportunity to express their thoughts and feelings about an impending examination would enhance test performance," says Sian Beilock, associate professor in psychology, in a UChicago news release.

Students were told that the exam would be videotaped and reviewed by math teachers.

Beilock and her colleagues tested the premise that just one experience of writing immediately before a test would be sufficient to enhance confidence and boost test scores.

For the research, 20 college students were given two short math tests. On the first test, they were instructed to "do their best." Before the second test, however, researchers upped the ante. Students were told that those who performed well would receive money and that their results would be part of a team effort. They were also informed that the exam process would be videotaped and reviewed by math teachers.

Before the second test, half of the students were given 10 minutes to write about their feelings about the upcoming test. The other students (the control group) were told to sit quietly.

"The expressive writing group performed significantly better than the control group," the authors write. "Control participants 'choked under pressure,' showing a 12 percent accuracy drop from pre-test to post-test, whereas students who expressed their thoughts before the high-pressure test showed a statistically significant five percent math accuracy improvement."

Beilock's research was published in the January 14, 2011 issue of *Science*. She is a leading expert on how the brain reacts to stress, and author of *Choke: What the Secrets of the Brain Reveal About Getting It Right When You Have To*.

Strategy Number Two: Meditation

Poorly performing students from a California middle school improved their scores in English and math as a result of participation in a Transcendental Meditation® program. Transcendental Meditation (TM) is a mantra-style meditative technique that does not involve any change in beliefs, values, religion or lifestyle. The research was conducted by the Maharishi University of Management (MUM), with news of the study released in November 2011.

Ninety-seven percent of the 189 students participating in the study were from racial and ethnic minority groups. 125 of them meditated and 64 others were in the control group. The students practiced twice daily for three months before being re-assessed for changes in academic achievement as measured by the California Standards Tests.

Participating students voluntarily chose the meditation program from a variety of Quiet Time program activities.

"The results of the study provide support for a recent trend in education focusing on student mind/body development for academic achievement," said Dr. Ronald Zigler, study co-author and associate professor at Penn State Abington. "We need more programs of this kind implemented into our nation's public schools, with further evaluation efforts."

Teachers may have benefitted from the program as much or more than the students. The news release from MUM states: "Faculty surveyed as part of the project reported the Quiet Time/Transcendental Meditation program to be a valuable addition to the school. They reported the students to be calmer, happier, and less hyperactive, with an increased ability to focus on schoolwork. In terms of the school environment, faculty reported less (sic) student fights, less abusive language and an overall more relaxed and calm atmosphere since implementation of the program."

> *Students who practiced meditation were calmer, happier and more focused.*

Meditation techniques designed to improve focus, concentration and relaxation, such as TM, Mindfulness, Zen training or Open Focus™, tend to decrease arousal by lowering breath and heart rates and increasing brain integration and coherence.

Strategy Number Three: Belonging Exercises

Stanford University psychologists designed a 60-minute exercise that helps black and minority students overcome concerns that they won't fit into the college environment.

"We all experience small slights and criticisms in coming to a new school" says Greg Walton, an assistant professor of psychology whose research on the exercise was published in the March 18, 2011 edition of *Science*. "Being a member of a minority group can make those events have a larger meaning," he adds. "When your group is in the minority, being rejected by a classmate or having a teacher say something negative to you could seem like proof that you don't belong, and maybe evidence that your group doesn't belong, either. That feeling could lead you to work less hard and ultimately do less well."

Walton split 90 second-semester freshmen into "treatment" and "control" groups. Approximately half of the students in each group were either black or Caucasian. The treatment group read essays written by senior students of varying races and ethnicities that described the challenges they experienced fitting in during their first year in college. While all reported some difficulties, they explained how things improved for them over time. The control group read about other experiences unrelated to a sense of belonging.

The treatment group reported half as many visits to their doctors, and more of them were at the top of their graduating class.

Treatment group subjects were then asked to write essays about why they thought the older college students' experiences changed. The researchers asked them to illustrate their essays with stories of their own lives, and then rewrite their essays into speeches that would be videotaped and could be shown to future students. The point was to have the test subjects internalize and personalize the idea that adjustments are difficult for everyone.

Black students in the "treatment" group reported a greater sense of belonging and happiness as they were followed throughout their university careers. The exercise had no discernible effect on the Caucasian students.

The research paper by Walton and Professor Geoffrey Cohen reports that the grade point averages of black students who participated in the exercise went up by almost one-third of a grade between their sophomore and senior years. And 22 percent of those students landed in the top 25 percent of their graduating class, while only about five percent of black students who didn't participate in the exercise reached that level of achievement. At the same time, half of the black test subjects who didn't take part in the exercise were in the bottom 25 percent of their class. Only 33 percent of black students who went through the exercise did as poorly. The "treatment" group also reported half as many visits to their doctors compared with the control group.

Conclusion

Each of the above-mentioned techniques is simple and unsurprising in a way. They don't offer some completely new way of being human but rather quantify what many of us have long known, and what school systems at all levels have been reluctant to acknowledge: that students are emotional beings like everyone else. People are driven by complex emotional and psychological needs that must be addressed in order for good learning to take place. Let's hope the excellent practices tested in the above studies: expressive writing, meditation and belonging exercises, are implemented at all levels of our education system.

Each nerve cell receives connections from other nerve cells at six sites called synapses. But here is an astonishing fact — there are about one million billion connections in the cortical sheet. If you were to count them, one connection (or synapse) per second, you would finish counting some thirty-two million years after you began. Another way of getting a feeling for the numbers of connections in this extraordinary structure is to consider that a large match-head's worth of your brain contains about a billion connections. Notice that I only mention counting connections. If we consider how connections might be variously combined, the number would be hyper-astronomical — on the order of ten followed by millions of zeros. (There are about ten followed by eighty zeros' worth of positively charged particles in the whole known universe!).

Gerald M. Edelman
Bright Air, Brilliant Fire: On the Matters of the Mind (1992)

Chapter 17

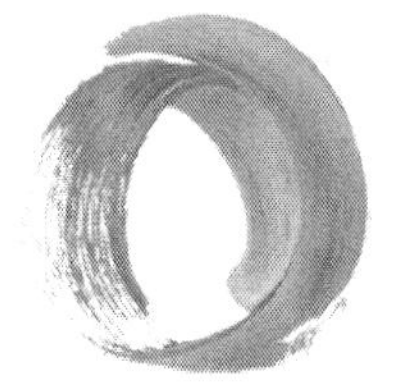

Hook Up Your Head:
Neurofeedback Renews Lives

Deborah DuSold was falling off chairs and walking into walls. She couldn't decide whether it was more important to do her nails or pay her bills. Given her high IQ and work as a molecular biologist, DuSold could certainly afford to lose a few brain cells and still function above normal, but this was nothing like normal. It was a nightmare. The nightmare lasted four long years, the result of a head injury DuSold sustained in a car accident. And despite having the best medical help available in her home state of Arizona, no one could give her any hope.

* * *

Paul Bruyere collapsed on the beach in Hawaii, his heart ready to burst from his chest, sweat streaming down his face. He was rushed to the hospital and diagnosed with — nothing. The high-powered businessman simply went back to work, hoping it wouldn't happen again. But the condition, later diagnosed as panic disorder, again brought him to his knees, gasping for air, this time on a golf course in Victoria, B.C. Panic Attack Syndrome is poorly understood. The condition has no cure.

* * *

A Los Angeles-based cameraman John Smith (not his real name) was hospitalized three times for depression. He dropped out of school and alienated friends because of his illness. Work as a cameraman in Hollywood was difficult to find because most days he couldn't bring himself to get out of bed. Smith was growing desperate.

* * *

Life for Deborah, Paul and John improved dramatically, thanks to a relatively new brain science technology – neurofeedback (NF). It has also helped many others suffering from a wide-range of conditions, including ADD/ADHD, migraine headaches, Obsessive Compulsive Disorder (OCD), alcohol addiction, cerebral palsy and epilepsy. Not only that, but neurofeedback works on so-called "normal" brains to enhance performance at work and play (many professional athletes use it).

NF is biofeedback for the brain, a high-tech process for training the brain to re-set its complex operating system for optimal functionality. This chapter will explore its origins, impressive claims and possible limitations.

Origins of Neurofeedback

In 1958, American research psychologist Joe Kamiya was the first scientist to discover that individuals could control their own brainwaves. The power of neurofeedback to change lives was discovered in the 1960s when researcher Barry Sterman discovered that cats could rapidly learn to produce a distinct brain rhythm associated with being calm, yet alert.

In a subsequent experiment for NASA, Sterman found that the cats he had previously trained in brainwave control were far less likely than other cats to experience seizures when exposed to toxic jet fuel. When Sterman tried neurofeedback with a woman who suffered from a severe seizure disorder, she became seizure-free after just three months of training. He went on to conduct at least two additional studies on epileptics that showed recovery rates of over 60 percent. His studies were replicated by independent laboratories and published in peer-reviewed journals.

Studies with epileptics showed recovery rates of over 60 percent.

Help for Addicts

American Eugene Peniston pioneered neurofeedback as a solution for addiction in the 1980s. Peniston used EEG-based biofeedback in conjunction with a 12-step program and had a remarkable success rate of 80 percent with men who were both addicted to alcohol *and* suffering from Post-Traumatic Stress Disorder (PTSD). His work was picked up by Bill Scott, an addictions counselor working on an alcohol-imbued native reserve in northern Minnesota.

Says Scott: "I thought his results sounded too good to be true but I sent two clients who had borderline personality disorder, alcoholism and PTSD, which is very difficult to treat, to a nearby program that used his protocol. These men were helped tremendously with only 30 sessions."

Scott and Peniston together conducted a study using neurofeedback in conjunction with a 12-step program that showed a 79 percent success rate with 24 chronic alcoholics. These results are in striking, almost inverse contrast to more common reports of relapse rates as high as 70 percent one year after treatment.

A 70 percent success rate with alcoholics one year post-treatment is astounding.

Scott subsequently helped to design a study (under the auspices of the UCLA Neuropsychiatric Institute) that demonstrated 77 percent abstinence for experimental subjects (12 months post-study), compared to 44 percent abstinence for controls.

Scott developed proprietary neurofeedback software in 2005 that is simple for the average person to use. BrainPaint™ turns EEG readings into stunningly beautiful, 3-D-like abstract patterns known as fractals that continuously morph in response to brain activity.

The Client Experience

What happens in a neurofeedback session? It depends on which of the many systems is being used. Generally speaking, the client is hooked up to an EEG machine with one or more sensors pasted to his scalp. In one of the more basic versions, the client is then shown a bar that represents a brainwave pattern from the EEG readout and asked to increase or decrease the levels on the bar by focusing on it (or to cause a red or green light to appear and stay on). With another system the client listens to music and then hears split-second static interruptions to let her know when her brain has gone off course. Some neurofeedback systems have users watch films or simple animations, which are interrupted with static. Such training is known as operant conditioning, the term for experiments in which subjects are rewarded for certain behaviors.

In the situations cited above, the "reward" is seeing the bar rise or fall, or noticing fewer interruptions in the audio or video feedback. Learning to control brainwaves is not usually achieved through effort, however; the brain does the learning and it's generally best to just relax and let that happen.

How *Exactly* Does it Work?

Most current neurofeedback systems provide feedback to strengthen some brainwave patterns while suppressing others. They can, for example, fine-tune the training to help the client develop greater access to emotions, or conversely, they can "turn down" emotional reactivity and increase the capacity for rational thinking. Using EEG readouts (linear representations of the electrical activity (hertz)

Brain training with NF can "turn up" or "turn down" emotional reactivity.

in the brain), these neurofeedback systems are based on clinical knowledge about how people experience various brainwave states.

For example, when the brain is in an alpha state it is relaxed, yet alert. The brain in theta is relaxed and in a pre-sleep mode. Beta brainwaves are used for everyday thinking and working, while gamma waves are present in high states of concentration and compassion. So, for example, if you report that you cannot shut off your thinking mind and are sleeping poorly, you may have an inability to shut off beta and enter theta. A neurofeedback device can then be set to adjust these ratios through the use of rewards when your brain goes to desired frequencies.

Some neurofeedback systems and practitioners do an assessment of what is going on in your brain as evidenced in an EEG reading before determining what training protocols to use, while other systems are more generic.

Neuropsychologist and former electrical engineer, Les Fehmi, has designed a generic neurofeedback system based on the premise that alpha wave synchronization across all lobes of the brain will benefit almost everyone in some way and will cause no harm. It is therefore designed to nudge your brain gently in that direction.

While some system developers, like Fehmi, hold strong beliefs about the efficacy of training for increased alpha wave production, others prefer to adjust the beta levels or SMR (sensory motor rhythm, a wave pattern discovered by Barry Sterman). Some clinicians believe in suppressing theta waves and others find them useful for evoking childhood memories, tranquilizing, and learning new information quickly. Others claim their equipment does not actually train for specific states but instead provides feedback on "turbulence" in the brain (e.g. the NeurOptimal System from Zengar Ltd). Another neurofeedback system – The Low Energy Neurofeedback System (LENS) – actually puts energy into the brain in the form of a very small electrical signal. The system, developed by Dr. Len Ochs in the early 1990s, uses weak electromagnetic fields to stimulate brainwave activity.

The challenge for both understanding neurofeedback and for its acceptance as a mainstream treatment for the many conditions it may help is that, as meditation teacher and neuroscience researcher Shinzen Young points out, "there is no coherent theory or body of knowledge as to what elements are critical, necessary and sufficient to evoke beneficial transformation."

Extraordinary results using entirely different systems are difficult to understand.

Practitioners and clients alike report extraordinary results using systems that operate on entirely different premises. Systems developed by Les Fehmi (ns500), Valdene Brown (NeurOptimal) and Len Ochs (LENS) have virtually nothing in common except for the fact that they stimulate the brain to behave in new ways. Even when the systems are essentially of the same type they often train the brain in different directions; for example Les Fehmi's system trains for synchronous alpha, while other systems train for beta, and still others for theta or a theta/alpha combination (which has been demonstrated to be a highly effective treatment for addictions and post-traumatic stress disorder (PTSD).

As Stephen Larsen, author of the excellent, LENS-favoring book, *The Healing Power of Neurofeedback*, says, "What is going on here?

"Positive clinical results have been obtained by training every range from theta to beta, including the vaunted alpha and SMR ranges, all of which have their adherents," notes Larsen, a psychology professor at the State University of New York, Ulster. "The only analogies that come to mind involve blind men and elephants, or spiritual sayings like, 'there are many paths to the one truth.'"

Larsen posits, "One possible reason for the success of this therapy is that we are training the student better to…control the way he/she focuses and deploys his/her attention."

Any current explanation of how NF works is bound to be simplistic and will probably be proved wrong in time. NF is based on EEG technology and EEGs are an imprecise and limited measurement of what is going on in the brain at any given time. In addition, while NF developers tend to present brain activity in simplistic ways in order to make the information more accessible to clients/patients (e.g. "you have too much beta") it is a fact that there is never just one kind of brainwave happening in the brain at any given time.

Is There a "Best" Neurofeedback System?
It is challenging for those who want to try neurofeedback to determine what approach or system would be best. Some systems are promoted as aids to overall happiness or peak performance while others claim to train for a wide variety of ailments (e.g. head injury, ADD or PTSD). It seems, on the face of it, fairly easy to understand what some systems do and how they do it, while other systems are too technical for the layperson to understand.

It may be helpful to consult with professionals in the field before making a decision on what system to try. There are health professionals (neuropsychologists, for example) who have presumably surveyed the various systems and selected those they feel will serve a multitude of clients best. But note that not all psychologists practice neurofeedback nor are they all well informed. Neuropsychologist Karen Shue, who practices neurofeedback at her clinic in Toronto, witnessed dismissive rudeness in an online professional forum when a fellow professional asked about the training. She notes: "I have seen in other places as well that without being familiar with the literature or techniques, physicians and psychologists are happy to express opinions on the (lack of) usefulness of NF for any number of conditions when asked by their clients/patients."

The average consumer is severely challenged when trying to buy an appropriate NF system for home use.

There are also many non-licensed practitioners of neurofeedback. Some of these have invested heavily in certain systems; there's one system that costs around $50,000 (most are far less). The practitioner may have trained only with the manufacturer of the system they purchased; they may not have shopped around and compared systems, and they may not have a wide knowledge base.

To complicate matters, system developers are often proprietary about the science behind their systems, wanting to keep their "secret sauce" from competitors. Therefore, the hope of moving this brain-enhancing tool known as NF into mainstream use is slim at present.

It must also be said that brain function is incredibly complex and science is just beginning to understand the brain and how to influence it. Discoveries take time to reach commercialization and some products currently on the market seem quite primitive compared to others. Sorting out the science from the marketing hype and making a well-informed purchase decision is challenging, to say the least.

Home-based or Via Professionals?

Deborah DuSold was so thrilled with the results of her neurofeedback training that she decided to open a clinic – MindWorks Studio LLC – in Tucson, where she offered NF along with massage therapy and nutritional counseling. Unfortunately, the lack of support from insurance companies for the neurofeedback training (along with the recession) made the cost prohibitive for many clients, and the clinic closed last year after five years of service to the community.

DuSold purchased several NF systems from a variety of manufacturers and hired people trained in their use. She has developed a significant knowledge base concerning which systems work best for various types of problems and would sometimes move a client to a second system when the benefits that can be derived from the first had been achieved.

It is possible to have negative reactions, such as panic attacks.

While DuSold did provide some systems to clients for home use, she feels strongly that most people benefit from working with a skilled practitioner. "It is possible to have negative reactions, such as triggering PTSD or panic attack," she explains. "I have also come to see the benefit of good counseling along with neurofeedback. People came to our clinic with many complex issues. A person might present as wanting peak performance but in fact have raging OCD. I wouldn't start doing neurofeedback on anyone without an assessment. This is serious stuff. While it's not dangerous you have to be careful."

This writer has undertaken neurofeedback brain training using both professional support and home-based systems. It is my opinion that both options are valid, depending on one's goals and current state of mental health. Users must keep in mind, however, that this is a buyer beware market, and that a consult with a knowledgeable professional may indeed be helpful. Further, if emotional material arises as a result of brain training, it may be helpful to know that this isn't unusual and may be part of the healing path. Again, however, a consult with a qualified professional can be a wise choice.

The Cerebral Palsy Connection

Corrine Fournier, a research scientist at a major French aeronautics company, discovered NF by accident. "I was browsing through a bookstore when I came across Jim Robbins' book, *A Symphony in the Brain*. On the back cover it claimed that NF helps autism and epilepsy, while also improving the performance of golf players and opera singers. I read it and became fascinated."

Fournier was so fascinated that she went on to establish a private practice using the NeurOptimal system. She also trains practitioners in its use, and has written a book on the subject, *Le Neurofeedback Dynamique* (available in French only) with her husband, Pierre Bohn.

About two-thirds of Fournier's clients are severely disabled with cerebral palsy. "They have lesions in their brains but the regulatory mechanisms still work and brain plasticity (the ability of the brain to create new connections at the cellular level) also exists," she explains.

Fournier trained a 17-year-old with cerebral palsy who wasn't able to pass an object from one hand to the other. After just a few sessions he mastered the task. He also learned to differentiate what he was eating. Fournier explains: "Initially, if an apple fell on the grass and he picked it up with grass on it, he would eat the grass, too. At the end of a session I gave him some little tomatoes and he dropped them, picked them up all covered with grass and carefully removed the grass before he ate them. His mother could hardly believe it."

A Course of Training

While anecdotal stories of near-miraculous results from neurofeedback abound, practitioners say that not everyone will benefit. "It typically takes about six sessions to know whether it is making any difference," notes Susan Cheshire Brown, one of the creators of the NeurOptimal system. "But it is not uncommon for improvements to be noted after just one to three sessions."

Cheshire Brown adds that when the brain self-corrects, people see improvements that allow them to be the best they can be. "Clearly the changes will be different for a professional athlete than they will be for a child with ADD or autism."

Paul Bruyere, the gentleman with panic disorder found that brain training with neurofeedback calmed his Type A personality: "I was always in a hurry to do everything and the neurofeedback calmed me right down. I noticed that I was playing golf a lot better too and I couldn't attribute it to anything except my new found calmer attitude."

John Smith came out of his depression, found work and is now a huge fan of neurofeedback.

Deborah DuSold, Paul Bruyere and John Smith were each helped by neurofeedback systems that operate in entirely different ways. While these success stories are impressive indeed, it will take some time before neurofeedback is thoroughly understood. In the meantime, anyone considering this option needs to be both open-minded and cautious.

*Lovers and madmen have
such seething brains,
such shaping fantasies,
that apprehend more than
cool reason ever comprehends.*
        William Shakespeare

Chapter 18

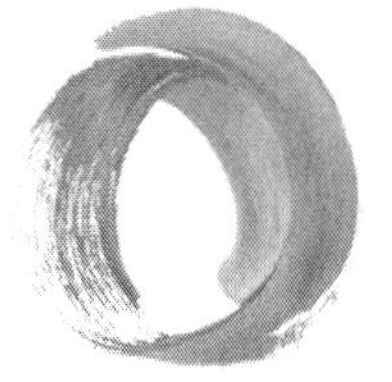

Eat Berries, Reduce Parkinson's Risk

People who eat berries regularly may substantially lower their risk of developing Parkinson's disease, according to research from the Harvard School of Public Health in Boston.

There is no known cure for Parkinson's, a neurological disorder that starts in the substantia nigra, an area of the brain responsible for the production of dopamine. A "feel-good" neurotransmitter, dopamine helps people to focus attention and enjoy pleasurable physical experiences. Dopamine also helps control muscles and movement, while its depletion leads to the characteristic motor symptoms (tremors, shuffling gate, loss of balance) that beset Parkinson's patients. The disease, which is generally found in people over 50, is one of the most common neurological disorders; it cuts across ethnic lines and affects approximately one in 100 people.

Flavonoids (also known as bioflavonoids), a group of chemical compounds found in fruits and vegetables, are the key to risk reduction. Also known as vitamin P and citrin, flavonoids are present in grapes, chocolate, apples and citrus fruits, in addition to being present in berries. They support visual acuity as well as having anti-inflammatory and anti-viral properties.

The Harvard study, recently released by the American Academy of Neurology, involved over 49,000 men and more than 80,000 women who were followed for 20 to 22 years. Researchers calculated each participant's consumption of flavonoids and analyzed the association between their intake and the risk of developing Parkinson's disease.

The results, which are impressive, differed between men and women. In men, those in the top 20 percent of bioflavonoid consumption were 40 percent less likely to develop the disease than the 20 percent who consumed the least.

The case with women was more complex. Although there was no relationship between overall flavonoid consumption and the development of Parkinson's, when sub-classes of flavonoids were examined, regular consumption of anthocyanins, which are mainly derived from berries (bilberries, black raspberries and black currants are particularly good sources), were associated with lower risk of the disease in both women and men.

The study was presented at the American Academy of Neurology's 63rd Annual Meeting in Honolulu, in April 2011.

"This is the first study in humans to examine the association between flavonoids and risk of developing Parkinson's disease," said study author Xiang Gao, MD, Ph.D., with the Harvard School of Public Health. "Our findings suggest that flavonoids, specifically a group called anthocyanins, may have neuroprotective effects. If confirmed, flavonoids may be a natural and healthy way to reduce your risk of developing Parkinson's disease."

The best of artists

hath no thought to show,

which the rough stone

in its superfluous shell,

doth not include;

to break the marble spell,

is all the hand

that serves the brain can do.

Michelangelo

Chapter 19

The Brain-Enhancement Sleuth

Working like a detective and diagnosing brain deficits with the mind-set of a Sherlock Holmes, Donalee Markus doesn't miss a thing. The Highland Park, IL-based clinical neuroscientist looks at your body language. Are you seated with both feet on the ground? Do you look up or down, to the right or left, when talking? Are you leaning or is your posture straight? How is your breathing?

Markus checks your hearing – from which direction do you hear a sound? She tests your peripheral vision, not as an ocular scientist but as a neurological sleuth. She does all this and more, before determining what kind of a learner you are. Are you a Left-to-Righter who sticks rigidly to systems? Or are you a Bottom Liner with a need for definite answers and guarantees? Can you consciously visualize your goals and determine what steps are necessary in order to achieve them? Can you, after experiencing failure, assess how you might in future adjust your actions to better meet those goals or new ones?

Markus doesn't determine your learning style and needs by asking how you see yourself (after all, you may not be aware of your deficits because you have compensated for them for so long); it's her sleuthing that gives her the information she needs.

Not only does Markus know the right questions to ask, she also knows how to address specific learning deficits with great precision; she has, in fact, invented thousands of ways to help people have better-functioning brains.

Markus' sleuthing helps her to determine what's going on (or not) in your brain.

Markus is a pioneer in brain plasticity, clinical research and cognitive tool development. More than 30 years ago she met with stunned silence when she declared, along with her then-mentor, Reueven Feuerstein, that the brain is malleable and can change at any age. "Feuerstein is the father of teachable intelligence," notes Markus. "And I am the Sherlock Holmes of maximizing intelligence and the capacity to learn."

Many corporations have hired Markus to get their staff thinking more creatively and to become better problem solvers, including NASA, where she worked with hundreds of scientists, including the top physicist and head engineer responsible for designing spacecraft.

How did Markus help the NASA scientists? She created the NASA Critical Thinking Game, which employs a series of complex geometric puzzles that are presented to the player in progressive steps. The game enhances critical thinking skills, working mental muscles in part-whole relationships and inductive and deductive reasoning.

Puzzles are, in fact, the primary learning tool for all of Markus' clients. With the help of a visual artist, she has created almost 20,000 puzzles that address different cognitive deficits, catalyze creativity, reduce stress and strengthen critical thinking skills.

Over 20,000 puzzles have been created by Markus to address specific cognitive deficits.

Puzzles "provide mild doses of confusion," explained Markus in an interview with BetterBrainBetterLife.com. "They're designed to challenge perspectives, expose weaknesses in cognition and strengthen perceptual skills. They provide a whole brain workout, clearing out the tendency to fall back into default thinking." Since they are a strictly visual form of challenge, the puzzles are also free of linguistic, class and cultural bias.

In addition to smart "normal" people who want to address deficits that limit them in life (e.g. the artist who can't balance a checkbook or the CEO who has poor emotional intelligence skills), Markus helps those with mild and traumatic brain injuries, learning disabilities, stroke, ADD and behavioral problems. Children and adolescents in her Learning How to Learn program develop better test-taking skills, improved study habits and increased creativity.

Clients who are fortunate enough to attend Markus' clinic in suburban Chicago visit her office once or twice a week and leave with about five hours of homework in the form of puzzles. It generally takes about 18 hours of cognitive intervention for clients with traumatic brain injuries to report improved sleep, less dizziness and improved depth perception. After 54 to 72 hours of treatment they report dramatic improvements in organizational skills, multitasking, self-confidence and tolerance for stress. Those on the normally healthy end of the spectrum may improve much faster.

Those with traumatic brain injury report improved sleep, less dizziness and better depth perception.

"My clients report that the DSM (Designs for Strong Minds) training program helps them deal with problems more objectively. They notice that they're able to assess new information 'on the fly' and adjust their behavior to achieve the results they want. They'll even learn to change their plans when their original objectives no longer appear feasible. This implies that they have learned to make better use of their working memories."

By taking advantage of the Internet, Markus makes her puzzle work available to everyone, albeit without the benefit of a diagnosis that pinpoints your exact cognitive needs. Her main website is: www.designsforstrongminds.com, and the game-specific site is offered online for a fee at: www.dsmexercises.com. Here you'll find the puzzles Markus created for NASA scientists, in addition to two other puzzle types.

Another great "take anywhere" option is Markus' iPhone app, known as Strong Mind Puzzles. "I wrote this app to address frontal lobe imbalance, which is the problem experienced by the largest number of people," she says. The game requires the user to correct pre-set errors on a grid of designs and involves distinguishing sameness or differences, or combinations of the two. Complexity increases with each level, for eight levels of complexity with thousands of individual puzzles. For a mere $1.99, the game is accessible to children and adults and offers hours of brain-enriching fun.

Markus' iPhone app addresses the problem experienced by the largest number of people: frontal lobe imbalance.

Business people who want to get the cognitive jump on the competition will also want to check out Donalee Markus' book *Retrain Your Business Brain*, published by Dearborn, and now in its seventh edition.

It's exciting to know that the same know-how that created better business thinkers for companies and institutions like Encyclopedia Britannica, Los Alamos National Laboratory and Coopers and Lybrand is also available to the rest of us. This is very much a "real world" book, designed to give all kinds of thinkers the opportunity to retrain their thought processes to align with the realities of a faster-moving, more complex world.

It takes a great brain to help other great brains (as well as the lesser-endowed among us) to be more than we thought possible. That Donalee Markus helps such a wide range of individuals – from a girl born with half a brain to the top physicist at NASA – attests to the power of the learning tools she has created. Her sleuthing pays off time and again in better functioning brains and happier individuals.

*The evolution of the brain
not only overshot the needs
of prehistoric man,
it is the only example
of evolution providing a species
with an organ which it does not
know how to use.*

Arthur Koestler

Chapter 20

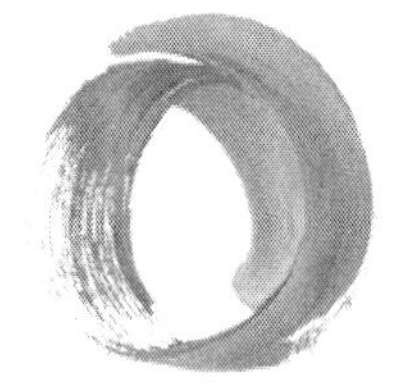

The Seeing Brain:
Rewiring for the Blind?

We tend to think that fixing "broken" things is intrinsically positive, especially when it comes to our bodies. Just imagine if the blind could see and the deaf could hear!

This chapter looks at the concept of brain plasticity with respect to the visual cortex. There is some fascinating research from different sources that shows what a brave new world we are entering, a world where we simply rewire the brains of the blind and – voila – we have a miracle.

But…is it really that simple?

American neurobiologist Paul Bach-y-Rita introduced the concept of neuroplasticity – the ability of the brain to change in response to experience – in the mid-1960s but it was many years before the idea gained wide acceptance.

Bach-y-Rita determined that we see with our brain, not our eyes. He was one of the first scientists to question localization (the idea that areas of the brain are hardwired for specific functions).

According to *The Brain That Changes Itself*, (a must-read book by psychiatrist Norman Doidge), Bach-y-Rita was working with a team, "that was studying how vision worked by measuring with electrodes the electrical discharge from the visual processing area of a cat's brain. The team fully expected that when they showed the cat an image, the electrode in its visual processing area would set off an electric spike, showing it was processing that image. And it did. But when the cat's paw was accidentally stroked, the visual area also fired, indicating that it was processing touch as well. And they found that the visual area was also active when the cat heard sounds."

The fact that the visual, auditory and sensory cortices all have similar processing structures was discovered by American neuroscientist Vernon Mountcastle of Johns Hopkins University and taken up by Bach-y-Rita, who published hundreds of articles and wrote several books on the subject.

In hindsight, the brain's ability to use the real estate in one region (say the auditory cortex) when another region needs more than usual power seems like a "no brainer." It's difficult to believe that no one prior to the 20th century noted that those with visual impairment tended to develop keener senses of touch, hearing and smell, or that those without hearing tended to have keener vision. Indeed, in the 1820s French physician and anatomist Marie-Jean-Pierre Flourens showed that the brain could reorganize itself. Such is the nature of human learning – one step forward and two steps back. But today, modern neuroimaging technologies have made such knowledge incontrovertible, for we can now see in real time where and how specific areas of the brain respond to stimuli.

Efforts to understand the precise nature of the plasticity of the brain in general and the visual cortex in particular continue today and a recent publication in the *Proceedings of the National Academy of Sciences* is a case in point. Researchers from the University of Montreal's Saint-Justine Hospital Research Centre, led by Dr. Olivier Collignon, recently published a study that compared the brain activity of people who can see with that of others who were born blind. The research was undertaken in collaboration with Dr. Franco Lepore of the Centre for Research in Neuropsychology and Cognition at the University of Montreal.

> *What would the brain's organizational structure for visual processing look like in people who have never seen?*

Collignon told BetterBrainBetterLife.com that the main objective of the research was to see if the organizational structure for visual processing evident in sighted people would be maintained in those who had never used these structures for vision. "We know that the occipital region is highly organized and processes different kinds of visual information in different areas," explains Collignon. "There is one area for movement, another for face recognition and another for spatial orientation. Would we find such organization in the occipital cortex of the congenitally blind?"

The researchers worked with 11 individuals who were born blind and 11 who were sighted. Their brain activity was analyzed via MRI scanning while they listened to a series of tones. "The results demonstrate the brain's amazing plasticity," Collignon said. "We learned that when a blind person processes spatial sounds they use the exact same region that sighted people use to make spatial distinctions with their eyes. So the region maintains the ability to process spatially but shifts to another sense modality if (it has been) deprived of vision since birth."

Gaining his sight made one man, blind since birth, very unhappy.

Whereas in Collignon's experiment the visual cortex was used to process sounds, another experiment on ferrets showed that the auditory cortex can rewire itself to process visual information. According to Doidge:

All reasonable doubt that the senses can be rewired was recently put to rest in one of the most amazing plasticity experiments of our time…Mriganka Sur, a neuroscientist, surgically rewired the brain of a very young ferret. Normally the optic nerves run from the eyes to the visual cortex but Sur surgically redirected the optic nerves from the ferret's visual cortex to its auditory cortex and discovered that the ferret learned to see. Using electrodes inserted into the ferret's brain, Sur proved that when the ferret was seeing, the neurons in its auditory cortex were firing and doing (sic) the visual process. The auditory cortex…had rewired itself so that it had the structure of the visual cortex. Though the ferrets that had this surgery did not have 20/20 vision, they had about a third of that, or 20/60 – no worse than some people who wear eyeglasses.

Other interesting research on the visual cortex has shown that restoring or instigating a person's vision isn't necessarily accompanied by the brain's ability to process the information received by the eyes. British scientists Professor Richard Gregory and J.G. Wallace published a fascinating paper in 1963 on a patient known as S.B. who had been blind since shortly after birth and had his vision restored at age 52. According to a paper published on Professor Gregory's website, S.B found much of what he saw confusing and overwhelming.

He changed from being an assertive and adventurous blind person into a sighted person with a profound lack of confidence, deriving almost no pleasure from his new sense of vision.

Similarly, auditory cortices may have a limited ability to process new sound information when deaf people receive cochlear implants. Other research from the University of Montreal by Dr. Lepore states:

All studies agree that congenitally deaf children implanted early in age when plasticity is greatest, perform better in open-speech perception tests than those who are implanted later. Furthermore, adults who have been profoundly deaf since birth are usually incapable of understanding speech from CI [cochlear implant] stimulation.

In conclusion, the brain most definitely rewires itself in response to experience, and it is well known that even into the senior years an individual's brain can make new neuronal connections. Nevertheless, it appears to be the case that once cross-modal accommodation has been made the brain may not be able to re-wire itself repeatedly, and that the earlier the rewiring is done, the more highly functioning it is apt to be. As shown in the cases discussed above, the phrase "Be careful what you wish for" bears consideration. Being bombarded with visual images or sounds that one can't make sense of seems like a kind of torture to me.

And men ought to know that from nothing else but thence [from the brain] comes joys, delights, laughter and sports, and sorrows, griefs, despondency, and lamentations. And by this, in an especial manner, we acquire wisdom and knowledge, and see and hear and know what are foul and what are fair, what are bad and what are good, what are sweet and what unsavory…And by the same organ we become mad and delirious, and fears and terrors assail us…All these things we endure from the brain, when it is not healthy…In these ways I am of the opinion that the brain exercises the greatest power in the man. This is the interpreter to us of those things which emanate from the air, when it [the brain] happens to be in a sound state.

Hippocrates

Chapter 21

Supplements for Your Brain?
Think First!

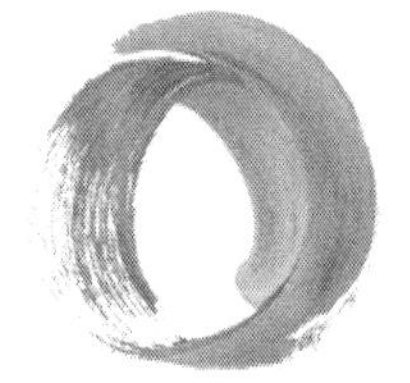

Southern California is surely the "health nut" capital of the world, a place where almost everyone strives to stay young, both physically and mentally. Pam Tarlow, an integrative pharmacist specializing in natural remedies, works in the high-pressure environment of a pharmacy in beautiful Santa Monica, where she is approached every day by anxious people seeking the proverbial "magic pill" to clear brain fog and improve memory. Can she help them? Well, yes…but it depends…

"Brain function is complicated," says Tarlow, "and normal brain function is built on the foundation of a healthy, functioning body, properly nourished and exercised. Beyond that, there are supplements that can help and typically you need to look at a few products to support various body systems."

Ask yourself these five essential questions if you're not thinking clearly or your memory seems to be in decline:

1. *When did I last eat and what did I eat?*
   "If you haven't eaten in more than two hours your blood sugar is probably low and this will affect your ability to think clearly," explains Tarlow. "For some people, just eating the wrong combination of foods (e.g. starches and sugar-based products) can result in fatigue and foggy-headedness."

2. *Could my adrenals be fatigued from too much stress?*
   Tarlow says that if you've been living with stress you may need to boost adrenal function through supplements (see suggestions below).

3. *Am I eating enough high-quality protein and thereby getting the amino acids I need?*
   "The body needs amino acids, derived from protein, to manufacture neurotransmitters (or brain chemicals)," says Tarlow. "Many people tell me they find their brain function improves with even a slight increase in protein consumption, especially after illness, injury or prolonged protein-restricted diets."

4. *Do I have circulatory problems?*
   "Blood vessel diseases, such as atherosclerosis, affect the brain as much as they do the heart and limbs," Tarlow points out.

5. *Might I be experiencing hormone imbalances?*
   "If you are having trouble with cognition, you may want to look at what is going on with various hormones. Thyroid,

adrenal (DHEA and cortisol) and sex hormones (estrogens, progesterone and testosterone) work together in a web-like fashion. They may significantly affect each other and influence brain and neurotransmitter function," explains Tarlow.

Should You Take Supplements?

Tarlow urges consumers to get professional advice on supplement use for cognition, and to beware of marketing hype: "Everyone's looking for the magic pill and all marketers know this. Every day I come across products that are badly misrepresented in advertisements and other forms of media. It's also important to note that supplements that help one person may not be optimal for another."

Here are Tarlow's recommendations for supplements that support brain function:

For adrenal support:

Vitamins C and **B complex** (especially B-5 pantothenic acid) and **adaptogenic herbs** (herbs that can help modulate physical, emotional and mental stress), such as rhodiola, ashwaganda, holy basil, various ginsengs and licorice.

Amino acids:

Tyrosine leads to production of the neurotransmitters L-dopa, dopamine, norepinephrine and epinephrine; it supports mood and mental clarity.

Acetyl-l-carnitine may increase production of the neurotransmitter acetylcholine, which is central to memory, attention, mental clarity, learning and mood support.

Choline in the form of GPC (Alpha-glycerophosphatidyl-choline) supports acetylcholine formation and stabilizes cell membranes for better cell-to-cell communication.

PS (Phosphatidylserine) also supports healthy cell membrane composition, allowing proper neurotransmitter function.

Other important supplements:

B vitamins are crucial for good cognitive performance. Production and utilization of neurotransmitters requires adequate B vitamins – especially B6 and B12. These can be supplied by a B complex or multi-vitamin. Our need for B vitamins may increase at different times in our lives, particularly while we're using certain medications, during times of high stress, and when consuming processed, nutrient-deficient foods.

Minerals work together with B vitamins, protein and other nutrients to support the brain. Zinc, magnesium and selenium can all play a crucial role.

Essential fatty acids (EFAs) (omega 3, 6 and 9 oils) benefit the entire body. In particular, the omega 3 fatty acid DHA supports the proper composition and shape of brain cell membranes so that neurons (brain cells) are better able to transmit and receive communication.

Use EFA products high in DHA from a trusted source that is labeled free of pesticides and heavy metals. Omega 3 DHA is available from fish and krill oil, and there is a vegan form from algae. Flax is a source of ALA, which is converted in our bodies to DHA as well as other omega 3 oils.

To enhance circulation:
One of the best things you can do for your circulatory system is to exercise. In addition, dietary antioxidants found in richly colored fruits and vegetables (including blueberries) are important.

Beneficial herbs such as gingko, grape seed extract, resveratrol, flavonoids, nattokinase and various forms of ginseng should only be taken on the advice of a qualified professional.

Hormones:
Hormone imbalances can only be addressed through medical testing and prescriptions from your doctor.

In closing, Tarlow says, "A comprehensive program designed to provide neurotransmitter support may be a good idea, and should be prescribed by a qualified health professional who will consider all factors related to your health, including current medications and supplements. If you are on medication for a health condition it is especially important to talk to your doctor and/or pharmacist."

*Aristotle was famous
for knowing everything.
He taught that the brain
exists merely to cool the blood
and is not involved in the
process of thinking. This is
true only of certain persons.*
Will Cuppy

Chapter 22

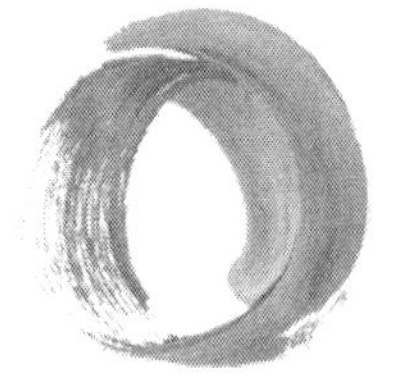

Money, Emotions and the Brain

If a friend offers to share a windfall with you, would you accept whatever she offered? What if your decision to reject the offer meant that neither of you would receive anything?

The Ultimatum game is an economics experiment that creates such a scenario. One person suggests to another how a pot of money should be split between them. The second player has the power to accept the offer or reject it.

The game gives rise to considerations of fairness, often accompanied by emotion. For instance, if you have $100 and only offer to give me $20, I might judge you as selfish and decide to forgo the offer, just to punish you.

How the Ultimatum game plays out in the brain is the subject of two recent studies, both of which reveal much about emotions.

The first study, published in *PLOS Biology*, was a collaboration between Sweden's Karolinska Institutet and the Stockholm School of Economics. Researchers scanned the brains of 35 subjects and those of a control group while they were playing the game. Previous research had suggested that the ability to analyze information and make decisions of a financial nature while playing the game were centered in the prefrontal cortex. While this may still be the case, the study in *PLOS Biology* revealed that a more primitive part of the brain, the amygdala, is also involved. This makes sense because the amygdala is the area responsible for emotional reactions that typically bypass the logical processing functions of the prefrontal cortex.

> *A Swedish study showed that the amygdala may be involved in making certain financial decisions. If so, logic may be circumvented.*

Researchers suppressed amygdala activity in some subjects with the anti-anxiety tranquilizer Oxazepam or a placebo while they played the game. They discovered that those with lowered amygdala activity were more likely to accept an unfair distribution of the money, despite the fact that they still considered the split to be inequitable. In the control group, the tendency to punish the player who suggested an unfair distribution of money was linked to increased activity in the amygdala. Men in the control group had stronger amygdala activity in response to perceived unfairness than women. Study subjects given the tranquilizer showed no gender differences.

While subjects in the Swedish study were often ruled by their emotional reactions to the Ultimatum game, another study, published in the April 2011 issue of *Frontiers in Decision*

Neuroscience, found that Buddhist meditators have developed skills that result in a very different experience of the game.

This research, conducted by Ulrich Kirk and Read Montague of the Human Neuroimaging Laboratory at Virginia Tech, and Jonathan Downar with the Neuropsychiatry Clinic and the Centre for Addiction and Mental Health at the University of Toronto, demonstrated that meditators have trained their brains to function more rationally and to make better choices in situations that carry an emotional charge.

The study showed that meditators make better choices when faced with situations that carry an emotional charge.

The researchers hypothesized that successful regulation of negative emotional reactions would lead to increased acceptance rates of unfair offers by the meditators. Mindfulness meditation teaches practitioners to pay attention to events in a non-judgmental manner. The behavioral results confirmed the hypothesis.

Twenty-six Buddhist meditators and 40 control subjects were recruited for the study, which, as with the Swedish study, monitored their brain processes with functional MRI (fMRI) scanning technology during game play. The brain scans showed that the controls had activation in the anterior insula, a region linked to the emotion of disgust, which plays a role in registering norm violations, mistrust and betrayal.

In the meditators, the anterior insula showed no significant activation for unfair offers; instead, meditators draw upon areas involved in interoception (the perception of body states) and attention to the present moment. While responders typically reject offers in which the proposer's share exceeds 80 percent of the total, meditators were more than twice as likely to accept those offers than were controls.

Perhaps the meditators didn't see any offer as unfair?

One might draw the inference, when comparing the two studies, that Buddhist meditation has a natural tranquilizing effect on the brain (and, indeed we report a study in Chapter 13, that claims meditation practice shrinks the amygdala). Whether or not that is true, the meditation techniques (including mindfulness) with which this author is familiar do not in any way dampen the *experience* of emotion. Rather, they give the practitioner the ability to fully allow emotions to arise in awareness, as body sensations, without being driven by them. A person without these skills is more likely to act impulsively on the basis of emotional triggers.

In the case of the Ultimatum game those emotions include disgust, and the behavioral outcome may well be to reject an offer perceived as unfair. The benefit to the meditator, in this instance, is that at least he or she ends up with something (e.g. $20) rather than nothing, and has not been discomfited by the behavior of others.

If you never change your mind,
why have one?

Edward de Bono

Chapter 23

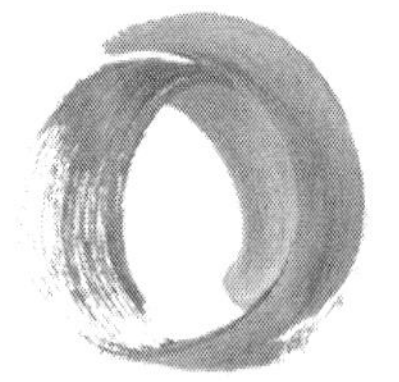

The Fearless Brain:
Amygdala Damage Erases Fear

When a woman who professes fear of snakes and spiders expresses a desire to touch and play with them, something must be off. And in the case of S.M., her amygdala, the almond-sized structure buried deep in the brain, is most definitely "off," destroyed by a rare condition known as Urbach-Wiethe disease.

In December 2010, the journal *Current Biology* published the results of a study on S.M. in which researchers at the University of Iowa (UI) found her unable to experience fear. While it has been known for some time that the amygdala plays a central role in fear reactions in animals, this was the first study to demonstrate that a functioning amygdala is essential for triggering a state of fear in humans.

S.M.'s disease caused calcification of the amygdala, beginning – it is estimated – at around the age of 10, the age at which she can recall her last experience of fear. Subsequent experiences that would have elicited fear in most or all people – including an incident where she was threatened with a knife – did not affect her at all.

In an interview with BetterBrainBetterLife.com, the study's lead author, Justin Feinstein, a doctoral student in clinical neuropsychology, said that S.M. experiences other emotions normally, including sadness, happiness, anger and grief.

Fear was the only emotion missing in this woman with a calcified amygdala.

"For a long time our field has had this notion that the amygdala is the central site for all emotions but the data does not seem to bear that out in patients with amygdala damage," explains Feinstein. "I've worked with a number of them and they are not emotionless. What we have stumbled upon is the fact that the amygdala seems to be extremely important in several things related to fear. It filters and processes sensory input from our environment and rapidly figures out if there is something going on that can impact our survival. It not only detects danger, but also initiates a rapid reaction in response to the danger. Fear is about survival and the amygdala is trying to keep us alive by helping us to steer clear of dangerous situations."

According to Feinstein, the fact that the amygdala is so necessary for our survival was demonstrated over 30 years ago when researcher Arthur Kling and colleagues lesioned the amygdalas in a group of wild monkeys and subsequently released them back into the wild. Within three weeks the majority of them had died, presumably because they lost their innate "radar" system that would have helped them to avoid danger.

As part of the UI study, S.M. was placed in close proximity to spiders and snakes, after telling researchers that she was afraid of them. "You couldn't pay me enough to get near them," notes Feinstein. "But she interacted with them with great curiosity. This comes back to the idea that the amygdala is navigating the fine balance between approach and avoidance."

Feinstein works with veterans who are experiencing post-traumatic stress disorder (PTSD). He hopes that the research findings from the study of S.M. (who has no amygdala and therefore no fear) can help lead to solutions for those with PTSD and related anxiety disorders, who have heightened amygdala activity. PTSD affects more than 7.7 million Americans, according to the National Institute of Mental Health. Feinstein says that one-third of combat soldiers returning from war zones will experience the disorder. Current treatments for PTSD include drugs that dampen amygdala activity, and psychotherapy.

*The mind can store
an estimated 100 trillion
bits of information —
compared with which
a computer's mere billions are
virtually amnesiac.*

Sharon Begley

Chapter 24

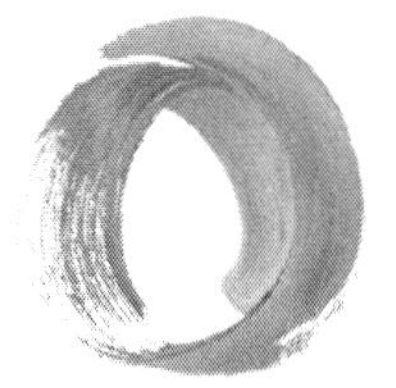

A "Brain" in the Ass? Poetry Says it All

This poem is of uncertain authorship. However, it has been attributed to American journalist Bert Leston Taylor, circa 1912. This version is from a lecture by W.R. Breneman, professor of zoology at Indiana University, Bloomington. Breneman helps us understand the poem with this brief introduction:

In Martinsville (Indiana), only a little more than 200 million years ago and 18 miles away, the dinosaurs were sovereign. They were interesting inasmuch as they were so strikingly physiological rather than psychological. Some flew like birds and others swam the oceans like huge sharks.

One of the largest of the dinosaurs actually had a brain, which weighted only a few ounces, whereas at the base of the spine there was an enlargement of the spinal cord, which weighed several pounds and was needed to coordinate the activities of its huge tail and derriere. This fact led an anonymous author to compose the following poem:

The Dinosaur: a Poem

Behold the mighty dinosaur
Famous in prehistoric lore
Not only for his weight and strength
But for his intellectual length
You will observe from its remains
The creature had two sets of brains
One in the head, the usual place,
The other at the spinal base.
Thus he could reason a priori
As well as a posteriori.
Since he could think without congestion
Upon both sides of any question,
No problem bothered him a whit:
He made both head and tail of it.
So wise was he, so wise and solemn,
Each thought filled just a spinal column.
If something slipped his forward mind
'Twas apprehended by the one behind.
And if in error he was caught
He had a saving afterthought.

Another poet, Don Marquis, proposed an appropriate addendum:

He failed to see the rocks ahead
That round them he might steer
And so he met the fate of all
Whose brains are in the rear.

*Have you tried
neuroxing papers?
It's a very easy and
cheap process.
You hold the page
in front of your eyes
and you let it go
through there
into the brain.
It's much better
than Xeroxing.*

Sydney Brenner

Chapter 25

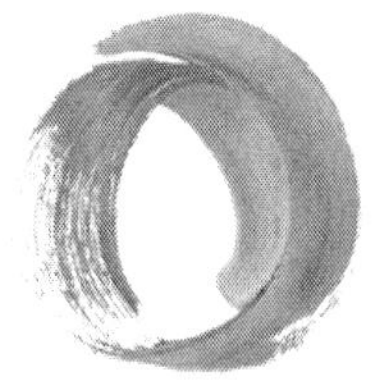

What We See: Vision, the Brain and an Open Mind

I had a startling experience with my eyesight after spending two days at a workshop with Dr. Les Fehmi learning how to broaden my attentional capacity. I was lying in bed in my darkened hotel room listening to tunes on my laptop. It was time to change the selection, so I turned on the light, sat up and looked at the screen without putting on my eyeglasses. The letters were quite blurry but then they came into focus just as if I had fine-tuned the focus on a pair of binoculars! This had never happened before.

The following day I brought my experience to the attention of Fehmi, originator of the Open Focus™ method of attentional training. While his training system has nothing to do with vision training, per se, he said that other users of the system have also experienced significant vision improvement.

Open Focus trains the mind to broaden awareness or focus by fostering increased alpha wave synchrony across the lobes of the brain. This gives rise to an experience of being relaxed, yet alert. This chapter is not about Open Focus per se (see Chapter Two: *Can You Imagine*) but rather about the possibility of improving vision via unconventional means. It was inspired by *Sight and Sensibility: The EcoPsychology of Perception*, by Laura Sewall, Ph.D.

Could a practiced "visualist" heighten the brain's ability to see, just as a pianist strengthens areas in the brain devoted to finger movements?

Why explore vision in a book on the brain? The visual system takes up approximately 30 percent of the brain's cortex, compared to eight percent for touch and three percent for hearing. We know the brain is plastic and that brain areas devoted to specific bodily skills can be strengthened or, if left unused, decay. If a professional pianist has super-strengthened brain areas devoted to finger movements, why cannot a "super-visualist" (my term for someone who practices eye movements and focusing) strengthen and improve vision?

The scientific method is based on observation, experimentation and repeated verification of results. It is also true that scientists are wrong much of the time, that they have persisted in beliefs that belie the facts (e.g. the belief that the brain cannot reorganize itself (plasticity) in response to experience), and that they, as typical human beings, are often not open to exploring the unexplainable, unexpected and unusual. Like people in other walks of life, scientists are sometimes more interested in maintaining the status quo than in discovering the full range of the possible. As you will see, vision science has not always been open to new ways of seeing.

Laura Sewall is a vision scientist who came to the study of vision partly as a result of experiencing a profound improvement in her vision via an unorthodox method. Having worn glasses for nearsightedness starting in her late teens, Sewall grew frustrated with the limitations her myopia imposed (like getting salt water stains on her glasses while kayaking) and began to study the Bates Method of Vision Improvement. She quickly noticed significant improvements in her vision – "I suddenly glimpsed sharp razor-like edges and neon colors…I could not believe my eyes….soon fabulous shapes and brilliant colors signaled to me, edges were sharp all the time… ."

Bates taught that the eye needs to relax and not "pull" objects to it.

One aspect of the Bates theory is that the eye needs to learn to relax and not pull objects to it, instead focusing both far and near, alternately, by performing specific exercises. Some of Bates' theories have been disproven, but what if this pioneer was actually on to something?

After her visual epiphany, Sewall traveled to Tanzania to study baboons in their natural habitat. It was here that she was further awakened to the possibilities inherent in the human visual system. She was amazed that her research partner, a Tanzanian scientist with years of experience on the savanna, could identify individual baboons from amongst three troops of 120, half a mile away.

By the time she got to Brown University's graduate school of vision science, Sewall had stopped doing most of the Bates exercises and gradually lost her superior visual acuity, because of too much computer work and reading. She writes:

> Despite the loss of my clear and inspired vision I continued my research. I read between the lines, asked many questions in carefully controlled labs and pieced together a developing story: The neural structure of the visual system changes when the attentional processes in the brain are activated. It was assumed by the researchers that this…occurred only during particular developmental stages in young animals. Among vision scientists the discussion of such fundamental change in the visual capacity of adult animals was apparently heretical. Questions posed in research seminars about structural changes in the adult visual system – questions that implied visual potential – were met with quick glances around the table and unsatisfying answers.

Sewall's search of the scientific literature showed that there were unanalyzed and unpublished data on structural changes in the visual cortex of animals that went well beyond the developmental stages. She became suspicious of scientific methods that ignored the outstanding in favor of the norm. "I learned that this kind of oversight is one of the classic limitations of Western scientific methodology. Like lies of omission, science names truth without reminding us that there is more to be revealed….Why, I wondered, did our research tradition focus on norms at the expense of identifying the great potential inherent in having…an exquisitely tuned human body?"

By participating as a subject in vision experiments on the absolute threshold (measurements of the capacities of the visual system), Sewall noted that she dimly saw lights that would be categorized by the researchers as "not seen," and that she would produce different results, indicating different levels of visual sensitivity depending on, "whether I'd had a cup of coffee before the experiment or too little sleep the night before. I also knew…that my overall visual sensitivity was noticeably greater after meditating….I began to realize that the absolute threshold for perception is relative." She also learned that the definition of "normal" or 20/20 vision defined by the Snellen Eye Chart was hardly a scientific measure. "I knew Snellen's story: He had established the standard for acuity by calling his assistant, who apparently had good vision, to the chart one day to measure what he could see from 20 feet away. And so it was that normal became normal."

Sewall became suspicious of scientific methods that ignored the outstanding in favour of the norm.

Sewall's perception of the difference in her visual acuity after meditation practice makes for a fascinating footnote in her book. "Theoretically, when the 'noise' – or spontaneous firings in the visual system – is temporarily quieted by meditating, the signal is rendered relatively more salient and is therefore more easily seen. This interpretation of the visual effects of meditation is derived from signal detection theory."

The above theory, and Sewall's personal experience, fit well with both Bates' concept of the need for the eye to relax and stop reaching for objects, and Fehmi's theories about why Open Focus (which is actually a type of meditation practice) might have been so effective in at least temporarily improving my eyesight on that one occasion. Could it be that

> *Can our brain more easily facilitate vision when we quiet the mind and broaden our focus?*

when we let go, broaden our focus and let the mind quiet, the brain can more easily do the job of helping our eyes? Is it possible that with training, we can become better at broadening focus and thus experience revived and enhanced sensory experience on many levels, not just vision?

Research on children and myopia appears to support this hypothesis. Dr. Justin Sherwin of the University of Cambridge conducted an analysis of eight studies on outdoor time and myopia in children and adolescents, representing 10,400 participants in total. He found that children who spent more time outside experienced considerably lower incidence of myopia than those who spent more time indoors. Sherwin surmised that one of the possible reasons for this difference is that children playing outdoors relax their gaze and also focus on distant objects more often.

The woman who taught Laura Sewall to dramatically improve her vision was the late Janet Goodrich, Ph.D. Her daughter, Carina Goodrich, herself a vision educator, has taken over her mother's business, which is based in Queensland, Australia. Carina Goodrich is also an author, having published *The Practical Guide to Natural Vision Improvement* in 2010.

Carina Goodrich says her mother wore glasses from age seven to 25, at which point she began to study the Bates Method along with the work of Margaret Corbett (a teacher of the Bates Method who also expanded on the work), in addition to Reichian Therapy (emotional/psychological healing based on the work of Austrian-American psychiatrist Wilhelm Reich). At age 27, Janet had the vision-related restriction removed from her driver's license and never wore glasses again.

After wearing glasses all her young life, Janet Goodrich no longer needed them.

Janet Goodrich consolidated the work of Bates, Corbett and Reich into her own method, which emphasized activities designed to decrease stress and increase relaxation in the visual system. She examined stress in the human body and its impact on eyesight. Goodrich trained instructors in her method and authored two books: *Natural Vision Improvement* and *How to Improve Your Child's Eyesight Naturally*.

Carina Goodrich notes that in Bates' era (1860–1931) the prevailing medical model was of the body as a kind of machine, with parts and systems generally considered as separate structures. At that time the eye was thought to work like a camera. "Bates, an ophthalmologist himself, headed in another direction and dared to suggest that the eyes are nothing like machines and that their ability to capture light and process it into clear images in the brain was dependent on much more than just the physical structure of the eyes. As our knowledge of the human brain and the effects of stress on every area of our health and well-being improves, Bates' theories about eyesight only increase in their sensibility."

Bates' work has been refined a great deal over the past almost 100 years, according to Carina Goodrich. "Yes, he was wrong about some things. For example, no one today would recommend looking directly at the sun. It is, however, the subsequent use and refinement of his work that helps to sort the wheat from the chaff. While his work still forms the basis of many things vision improvement therapists do today, they are usually quite different from what he originally proposed."

The brain adapts to the fact that you are doing extended close work and when you focus out it doesn't believe that you will stay there.

Developmental optometrist Dr. Leonard J. Press, the American Optometric Association's vision and learning specialist, and optometric director of the Vision and Learning Center in Fair Lawn, NJ, has also carefully considered Bates' contribution to vision science.

"Bates definitely made a contribution, primarily in his concept of learning to relax focus," says Press. "People who do sustained close work definitely have a shift of their resting focus inward. The brain adapts to the fact that you are doing extended close work and when you focus out it doesn't believe that you will stay there. So it holds on to extra tonus (slight continuous contraction of a muscle) for near vision, believing you will come back to it. Bates understood that by consciously putting yourself in a position of relaxation or distance focus, however you do it, you are going to limit the progression of nearsightedness. And vision science has proven him correct on this."

Many of Bates' original training techniques are crude compared to what is done by developmental optometrists today, notes Press. "That's where technology comes into play. There are many ways to reset focus to distance. For example, we can do this with accommodative rocking lenses, where one side stimulates focus and the other relaxes it."

Press finds that Bates' work has been elaborated

The curiosity of Bates, Goodrich and Sewall challenged what is possible in the human visual system.

into a holistic approach that is sometimes misleading. "I feel some of it is over-extrapolated," he says. He points to some Internet sites that present home-use vision training products as almost magical devices that will help everyone. "While they may be of some help to some people, they are not stand-alone solutions as the claims suggest." This writer agrees and urges caution, having researched several websites and tried some of the "one size fits all" equipment. Readers would do best to stick with the books mentioned in this chapter or visit a developmental optometrist.

Bates' curiosity and willingness to pay attention to the actual experience of his patients and try new methods to help them improve their vision is laudable. And Laura Sewall's thoughtful openness to new experience, combined with intellectual rigor have also contributed to our understanding of what is possible in the human visual system. Our world is made better by those who challenge the status quo. This often involves paying attention to the world around them *as it is,* unencumbered by received wisdom.

Laura Sewall's excellent book opens (and this chapter ends) with a quote from Søren Kierkegaard:

"If I were to wish for anything. I should not wish for wealth and power, but for the passionate sense of the potential, for the eye which, ever young and ardent, sees the possible."

*There can be no knowledge
without emotion. We may be
aware of a truth, yet until we
have felt its force, it is not ours.
To the cognition of the brain
must be added the experience
of the soul.*

Arnold Bennett

Chapter 26

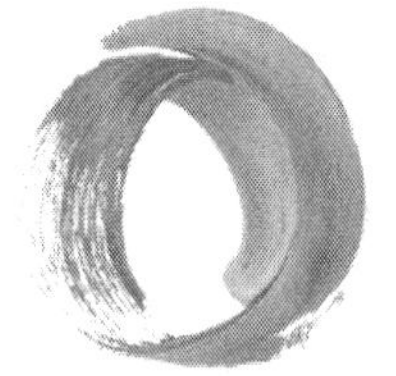

When You DON'T Want to Remember: Molecules of Memory Erasure Discovered

Given the chance to erase a traumatic memory, would you do it? What if erasing that one memory meant that memories of the days before the event would be erased as well?

Researchers Richard L. Huganir and Roger Clem of Johns Hopkins University School of Medicine have discovered that they can permanently delete fearful memories in rodents through molecular tinkering. In an interview with BetterBrainBetterLife.com Huganir explained that this discovery opens the door to effective drug therapy for permanent memory erasure.

Huganir and Clem used the research of Joseph Ledoux from New York University as a starting point. Ledoux had "magically," as Huganir puts it, "discovered that he could erase fearful memories in mice by making a slight change to a classic de-conditioning, or extinction, protocol. What we wanted to do was to discover how that erasure occurs at a molecular level."

It was well known that when researchers conditioned rodents to be afraid, the synapses in the amygdala (the fear center of the brain) became stronger and remained stronger for weeks. "What we discovered," notes Huganir, "is that after the initial fear conditioning, the properties of the stronger synapses totally changed. We found that a new receptor (a protein, the calcium-permeable AMPR) appears about 24 hours after the initial training and then within a few days totally disappears. We knew these receptors were unstable and could easily be removed, and so posited that if we did the memory extinction protocol during this sensitive period we might get total removal of the AMPR and erasure of the fearful memory.

That is exactly what happened – 100 percent of the time."

Currently, the erasure protocol needs to be implemented within 24 hours of the traumatic event.

Huganir and Clem are now working on finding drugs that will safely control and enhance the removal of calcium-permeable AMPRs. The challenges are many and include the need for drugs that will target specific memories only. One current limitation is that the protocol only works for recent memories and has to be implemented within a narrow window of opportunity (days, not weeks or years).

They're also studying whether the drugs work well on their own or if they work best in conjunction with behavioral therapy. "We're about a decade or more away from a drug-based solution," notes Huganir, "But the discovery of the mechanism for erasure is exciting and rewarding. We're especially hopeful that it will lead to effective treatment from debilitating fearful memories associated with war, rape and other traumatic events."

*How is it possible that a being
with such sensitive jewels as the
eyes, such enchanted musical
instruments as the ears, and
such a fabulous arabesque of
nerves as the brain can
experience itself as anything
less than a god?*

Alan Watts

Chapter 27

One Man's Magic Brain

Almost dying – twice – didn't get the better of Donald Parker, a man with a thread of magic running through his life that weaves suffering and success together in a remarkable pattern. Looking back, it seems miraculous that he survived at all.

Like all of us, Donald was born into an uncertain world. Unlike most, however, his mother took her life soon afterwards.

No one knows if this tragic loss triggered Donald's lifelong mental health problems and attention deficit hyperactivity disorder (ADHD) but school was a disaster for him. Moreover, his home life was very difficult. He saw his first psychiatrist at seven, began drinking socially at 14, and by the time he reached his 20s, was cross-addicted to alcohol, cocaine, heroin and methadone.

Not that it was all bleak. His father remarried when Donald was two, and he has always been close to his stepmother Mary, while greatly admiring his father, an actor and director. They encouraged his passion for magic, indulging him with expensive magic books and tricks as Christmas and birthday presents. By age 12, Donald was earning money performing at children's parties. Acting in his father's plays helped his performances come to life. In his late teens and early 20s he performed in nightclubs using birds, fire, flashy costumes and elements of dance to keep audiences enthralled. But the success proved illusory, as the years of substance abuse and inner turmoil took their toll. Work dried up and Donald coped poorly.

I was desperate for my next hit and decided to kill myself.

"By age 24 I was living on welfare in a dingy basement apartment, desperate for my next hit and I decided to kill myself," recalls Donald. "I had a large bottle of vodka and plenty of prescription drugs in my bathroom drawer, the remnants of failed attempts to treat my bipolar disorder. I took all the pills I could find and washed them down with straight vodka."

Donald's stepmother is an intuitive woman who cares deeply about him. She sensed in that moment that he was in grave danger and phoned his landlord, urging him to knock on Donald's door. When Donald didn't respond, the landlord told Mary not to worry. Undeterred, she called a friend and begged him to go over.

"Please, go to Donald's place now and if he doesn't answer break down the door! I know something is very wrong."

The friend found Donald unconscious on the floor and called 911. When he awoke from the coma three days later a fresh hell awaited him.

"For a week I was terror-stricken, not knowing who or where I was," he says. "I was hallucinating far beyond any drug I had ever taken."

After a full year of treatment Donald was clean, sober and psychologically stable, maybe for the first time ever. He embraced his new life, delving into philosophy and spirituality, studying motivational speakers, taking courses and learning about the power of the mind. Combining his love of magic with a desire to influence young people, Donald created a new act featuring magic, motivational messages and information about drug and alcohol abuse. He began in local high schools, eventually working with an agent who marketed the show to colleges and universities in Canada and the U.S.

"It was an amazing experience and a fabulous lifestyle," he notes. "Many kids told me what a profound effect the show had on their lives. And, I was in love with Susan. We lived together in Vancouver and were engaged to be married."

From out of his body, Donald could see the traffic backing up.

Corporate work was a lucrative sideline and it was on his way to one such event in Whistler, driving up the highway that snakes along the rugged shoreline north of Vancouver, that Donald's life changed again. The driver of an oncoming Ford Explorer fell asleep at the wheel and hit Donald's Jeep head on, jamming his face into the exploding air bag and shearing his brain against the bony interior of his skull.

Donald's consciousness suddenly seemed to leave his body and he had an out-of-body experience. He'd never been *above* a scene before; now he not only seemed to be higher than the mountains but also had a 360-degree view of everything, including the traffic backing up on the high-way. That his battered body was at the center of the scene was unknown to him at that point.

Donald was airlifted to Vancouver General Hospital, where he spent weeks in a painful physical recovery. He eventually tried to resume his performance career, but when clients complained that he was staring into space and almost falling off the stage, his agent fired him. It was the traumatic brain injury (TBI) that caused the blanking-out episodes and loss of balance. Inappropriate bursts of anger and out-of-proportion weepiness, also signs of TBI, alienated him from friends and family, and led to a break-up with Susan. Donald was exhausted and virtually housebound for five years. He even returned to drinking and soft drugs for a short while. But life had other plans for him, and the art of magic provided a new lease on his fragile existence.

"I had lots of time on my hands, so I got on the Internet and started buying new magic tricks and training videos. I was learning again and the parts of my brain that were dormant or damaged slowly came alive. I was having fun and the spin-off benefits were really exciting: my memory improved, as did my executive functioning and physical en-ergy. A year later I found a part-time job and returned to motivational speaking."

There is a broad body of research that backs up Donald's understanding of how learning new magic tricks enhanced his cognitive function. Neuroplasticity is the term used to describe the various ways the brain changes in response to environmental conditions (it was previously believed that substantial re-wiring of the adult brain was impossible). Dr. Jeffrey Schwartz co-author with Sharon Begley of *The Mind and the Brain*, says, "People can learn to change how their brain responds to circumstances by focusing their attention differently. Focus of attention influences how the brain responds to phenomena, and those changes leave physical traces that you can see with brain imaging."

Donald's brain has been through a tremendous amount of trauma: just one of the three major events in his life – losing his mother as an infant, extreme substance abuse, and head injuries sustained by the car accident – could have rendered him a lifelong victim of mental and emotional disorders. The magic lies in his brain's nine-lives ability to recover and form new connections that have helped him to thrive, as well as in the support he has received from loving family and friends.

How does Donald view his life's path, the interwoven aspects of suffering and success? "I'm happier now, at age 46, than I have ever been. I'm living a normal life again and I have a new love relationship."

Donald is a magician. He still performs the occasional show for children, beguiling them with skillful illusions: which hand, where's the ball? More importantly, he has transformed his losses into gains and found a way to be happy. That alone is magic enough for anyone's life.

I look forward to hearing from you with any comments you may have about this book, or to share your own experiences of mind and brain.

Please contact me at: paddy@betterbrainbetterlife.com. You can also visit www.betterbrainbetterlife.com to sign up for my newsletter, and to register for a copy of my next book on brain-enhancing technologies. I've been testing out these technologies for a few years now and you may be interested in what I am learning.

With Appreciation

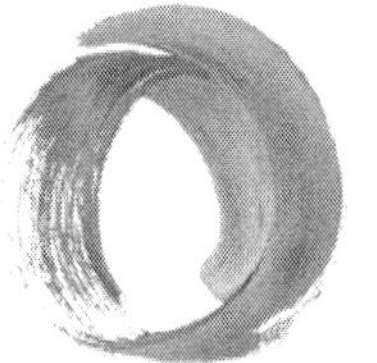

I heartily thank the researchers, clinicians and practitioners who spoke with me about their work, as well as Claudia Osborn and Donald Parker, who shared their harrowing life stories with me.

Medical writer Rosemary Frei generously contributed three articles to the BetterBrainBetterLife website. Two of the articles – *Back to the Cradle? Rocking the Brain to Sleep* and *Grow Your Brain's Memory Center* – have been included in this book. Thank you, Rosemary.

Integrative pharmacist, consultant, meditation and conscious-eating coach Pam Tarlow approved a rewrite of a previous article on her work, which appeared in www.betterbrainbetterlife.com. Thank you, Pam.

Chapters 20 and 25, on vision and the brain, were originally published in Envision magazine, a trade publication for which I am the editor-in-chief.

I extend my great appreciation to Raffaela Civello, a successful businesswoman who pinch-hits for me as an occasional (and very good) editor, strategist and all-round great friend. Our mothers have Alzheimer's disease, which brings us even closer.

My father, Gordon Jeffries and his wife, Violetta, and my mother Ethel Jeffries and her husband, Robert, have always encouraged me to be my self. This is a gift beyond words.

Finally, my spouse and fellow wordsmith, JoAnne Sommers, kindly edited this volume and has always encouraged me to follow my dreams. What a blessing!

Paddy Kamen

June 1, 2013

About the Author

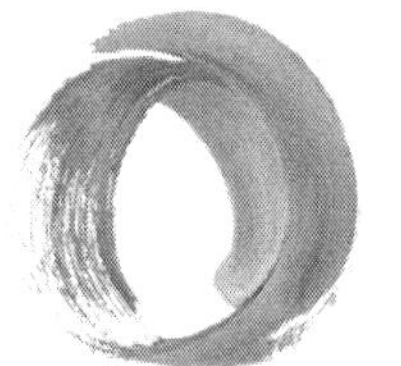

Paddy Kamen has been published in Canada's leading media, including the *Globe and Mail*, the *Toronto Star*, *Maclean's* magazine, and *Canadian Business* magazine. She lives in British Columbia, where she keeps pausing to notice what is around her, breathe in love and practice appreciation (especially on those grumpy, gloomy days).

Kamen enjoys her superb friends, and extended family of loving parents and brother, their spouses, her own spouse, three sons and their partners, and three grandsons (that's six more amazing men in our world!).

She can be reached at paddy@betterbrainbetterlife.com. Readers can get on her email list for notification of upcoming books by visiting: www.betterbrainbetterlife.com.

Index

Made in the USA
San Bernardino, CA
03 September 2013